The Cranial Nerves

The Cranial Nerves

Dominique Doyon

Kathlyn Marsot-Dupuch

Jean-Paul Francke

Translated from the French by Donald Schwartz

Illustrations by Guillaume Blanchet

Including additional illustrations by Frank H. Netter

Icon Learning Systems · Teterboro, New Jersey

FIRST ENGLISH EDITION, 2004

Published by Icon Learning Systems LLC, a subsidiary of MediMedia USA, Inc.
Originally published as *Nerfs crâniens. Anatomie, clinique, imagerie*
©**Masson, Paris, 2002**

This work has been published with the help of the French *Ministère de la Culture—Centre National du Livre*

FIRST ENGLISH EDITION

10 9 8 7 6 5 4 3 2 1

ISBN 1-929007-54-X
Library of Congress Catalog No.: 2003097821

NOTICE

Every effort has been taken to confirm the accuracy of the information presented and
to describe generally accepted practices. Neither the publisher no the authors can be held
responsible for errors or for any consequences arising from the use of the information
contained herein, and make no warranty, expressed or implied, with respect to the
contents of the publication.

Executive Editor: Paul Kelly
Editorial Director: Greg Otis
Managing Editor: Jennifer Surich
Director of Manufacturing: Mary Ellen Curry
Production Editing Manager: Stephanie Klein
Graphic Designer: Colleen Quinn
Digital Asset Manager: Karen Oswald

Binding and Printing by Printcrafters, Inc. Printed in Canada.
Composition and layout by Cenveo

Foreword

Since the beginning of his career, Dominique Doyon has shown an unrelenting interest in the imaging of the base of the skull and the cranial nerves. After having fully explored all the possibilities offered by conventional radiography and tomography, Dominique Doyon, neuroradiologist; Kathlyn Marsot-Dupuch, eye, ear, neck, and throat (EENT) specialist; Jean-Paul Francke, professor of anatomy; and their collaborators have become highly familiar with the most up-to-date techniques in computed axial tomography and MR image. In this book, the authors exhaustively discuss the different anatomic, physiologic, and pathologic aspects of the cranial nerves after first presenting a very useful chapter on some basic clinical aspects. This book will undoubtedly become a reference text for neurologists, neurosurgeons, ophthalmologists, surgeons working in EENT and stomatology, as well as for neuroradiologists. The quality of both the text and the illustrations promise to make it an excellent tool for students who will readily recognize the didactic prowess of the authors.

Henceforth, in complement to the information provided by physical diagnosis, modern imaging techniques allow physicians to follow cranial nerves almost completely along their pathways. Undoubtedly, these new techniques will ultimately benefit patients by allowing clinicians to forego invasive procedures.

Professor Gérard Said
Chief of Neurology
Bicêtre Hospital

Preface

The diagnoses of neuralgias and paralysis of the cranial nerves has been transformed by MR image (MRI). MRI analysis of the cranial nerves requires a thorough knowledge of the anatomy of these nerves from their origin to their ending, of the clinical features of these nerves, and finally, excellent radiologic technique. MRI allows clinicians to study the cranial nerves directly and to obtain excellent analytical precision in the three geometric planes; thus, it has become possible:

- To precisely locate the nuclei of these nerves at their origin or nerve-ending, as well as their pathway through the brain stem.
- To directly visualize the nerves in the intracranial pathway in the cisterna.
- To visualize the cranial nerves in the apertures or canals from which they enter or exit the skull; with modern-day reconstruction techniques, these openings are easily analyzed by computed axial tomography.
- To be able to analyze occasionally the intracranial pathways of these nerves from their endings to their origins.

The caliber of the nerves (ranging from 0.3 mm for the IV or the VI to 3.6 mm for the V nerve, according to Lang) explains the variability in their visibility; in addition, the IV and VI nerves are inconsistently visible.

Regarding study techniques, we emphasize the importance of obtaining images with excellent definition and a narrow study field (between 12 and 16 cm) as well as fine, 2- to 3- mm sections during weighted T1 spin echo sequences with and without gadolinium injection in at least 2 spatial planes with or without fat suppressed. Inframillimetric sequences during three-dimensional gradient echo in T2 or during rapid spinecho are essential for studying the cisternal portions of the nerves.

A study of the entire brain should be obtained when multiple sclerosis or other diffuse disorders are suspected.

When compression from a vascular loop is present, inframillimetric sequences are essential; study of the arteries during steal time after injection permits better assessment of the topography and the type of vessel involved.

Finally, radiography with inframillimetric sections permits excellent assessment of the bony structures of the temporal bone, the spheno-orbital and facial regions, the exit orifices of the cranial nerves, and the bony walls to look for calcifications, bone lysis, or an expansive process.

The vascular disorders (diabetes mellitus, hypertension, dissecting aneurysm) should not be neglected. These disorders often produce lesions in the cranial nerves, but the roles of these disorders are difficult to prove.

We hope that readers will continue to improve their ability to diagnose cranial nerve paralysis or neuralgia because they have better clinical and anatomic knowledge on the one hand and the possibilities offered by imaging on the other.

We thank Mrs. Isabelle Lemanissier for secretarial assistance and Christine Duchateau for critical review of the text.

CONTRIBUTORS

Farida Benoudiba, *Radiologist, Neuroradiology Unit, Bicêtre Hospital*

Marie-Germaine Bousser, *Professor of Neurology, Chief of Neurology Unit, Lariboisière Hospital, Paris*

Laurent Brunereau, *Professor of Radiology, Chief of Radiology Unit, Bretonneau Hospital, Tours*

Françoise Callonnec, *Staff Physician, Radiologist, Cancer Unit, Rouen*

André Chaÿs, *EENT Professor, Chief of EENT Unit, University Hospital, Reims*

Fernanda Curros-Doyon, *Radiologist, Fellow, Pediatric Radiology Unit, Bicêtre Hospital*

Florence Domengie, *Radiology Resident, Bretonneau Hospital, Tours*

Dominique Doyon, *Professor of Radiology, Neuroradiology Unit, Bicêtre Hospital*

Denis Ducreux, *Radiologist Fellow, Neuroradiology Unit, Bicêtre Hospital*

Monique Elmaleh-Bergès, *Radiologist, Radiology Unit, Robert Debré Hospital, Paris*

Jean-Paul Francke, *Professor of Anatomy, Anatomy Laboratory, Faculty of Medicine, Université du Droit et de la Santé, Lille*

Françoise Fuerxer, *Radiologist, Radiology Unit, Princesse-Grace Hospital, Monaco*

Marie Gayet-Delacroix, *Radiologist, Radiology Unit, Hôtel-Dieu Hospital, Nantes*

Patrice de Greslan, *Assistant, Neurology, Neurology Clinic, HIA Val de Grace, Paris*

Mouhoub Hadi-Rabia, *Former Radiologist, Neuroradiology Unit, Bicêtre Hospital*

Clément Iffenecker, *Former Radiologist, Neuroradiology Unit, Bicêtre Hospital*

Kathlyn Marsot-Dupuch, *Professor of the College of Medicine, Associate Chief of Neuroradiology Unit, Bicêtre Hospital*

Hervé Offret, *Professor of Ophthalmology, Chief of Ophthalmology Unit, Bicêtre Hospital*

Marie-Christine Petit-Lacour, *Chief Resident-Assistant, Neuroradiology Unit, Bicêtre Hospital*

Jean-Luc Poncet, *EENT, Chief of Service, HIA Val de Grâce, Paris*

Jean-Luc Sarrazin, *Professor of Radiology, Medical Imaging Service, American Hospital, and Neuroradiology Unit, Bicêtre Hospital*

Didier Soulié, *Radiologist, Former Specialist in the Hospitals of the Armies, Agen*

Jacques Thiébot, *Professor, Chief of Radiology Unit, Charles-Nicolle Hospital, Rouen*

Katayoun Vahedi, *Neurologist, Neurology Unit, Lariboisière Hospital, Paris*

Thierry Van Den Abbeele, *EENT Professor, Chief ENT Unit, Robert-Debré Hôspital Paris*

D. Doyon,
K. Marsot-Dupuch,
and J.P. Francke

Table of Contents

C H A P T E R *13*

The Sympathetic and Parasympathetic Nervous Systems of the Head and Neck 225

J.-L. Sarrazin, P. de Greslan, and J.-L. Poncet

Introduction

In the illustration, in addition to the real anatomic figures and schemas, we added 13 Frank H. Netter plates (one of which is for the cover); they are remarkably didactic and synthetic.

Below is the list with their reference pages:

0 : cranial nerve (motor and sensory distribution): schema plate (PL) 112 cover
1 : olfactory nerve (I): 2 schema PL 113, page 17
2 : optic nerve (II) (visual pathway): schema PL 114, page 23
3 : ciliary ganglion: schema PL 126, page 24
4 : oculomotor (II), trochlear (IV) and adbucens (VI) nerves: schema PL 115, page 36
5 : vagus nerve (X): schema PL 120, page 58
6 : accessory nerve (XI): schema PL 121, page 58
7 : hypoglossal nerve (XII): schema, PL 122, page 62
8 : taste pathways: schema PL 129 page 63
9 : autonomic nerves in neck, PL 129, page 231
10 : autonomic nerves in head, PL 125, page 232
11 : pterygopalatine and submandibular ganglia: schema PL 127, page 233
12 : otic ganglion: schema PL 128, page 234

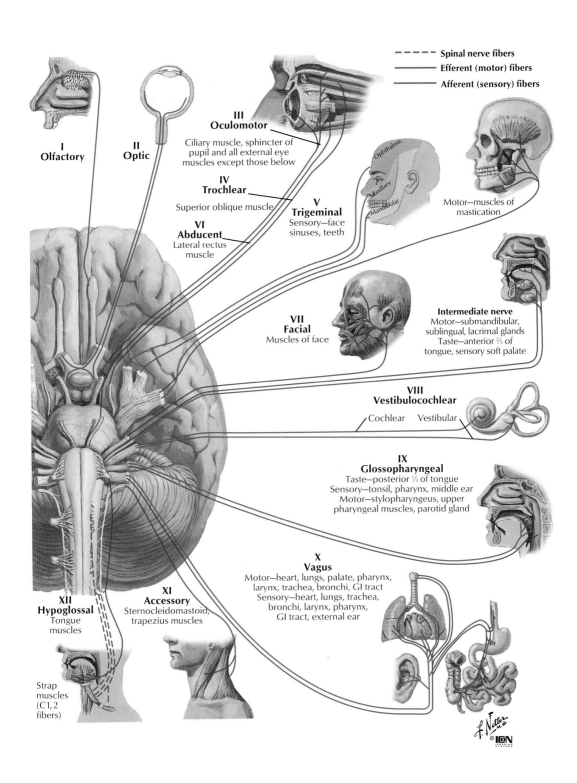

Spinal nerve fibers
Efferent (motor) fibers
Afferent (sensory) fibers

I
Olfactory

II
Optic

III
Oculomotor
Ciliary muscle, sphincter of
pupil and all external eye
muscles except those below

Ophthalmic
Maxillary
Mandibular

IV
Trochlear
Superior oblique muscle

VI
Abducent
Lateral rectus
muscle

V
Trigeminal
Sensory—face
sinuses, teeth

Motor—muscles of
mastication

VII
Facial
Muscles of face

Intermediate nerve
Motor—submandibular,
sublingual, lacrimal glands
Taste—anterior ⅔ of
tongue, sensory soft palate

VIII
Vestibulocochlear
Cochlear   Vestibular

IX
Glossopharyngeal
Taste—posterior ⅓ of tongue
Sensory—tonsil, pharynx, middle ear
Motor—stylopharyngeus, upper
pharyngeal muscles, parotid gland

X
Vagus
Motor—heart, lungs, palate, pharynx,
larynx, trachea, bronchi, GI tract
Sensory—heart, lungs, trachea,
bronchi, larynx, pharynx,
GI tract, external ear

XI
Accessory
Sternocleidomastoid,
trapezius muscles

XII
Hypoglossal
Tongue
muscles

Strap
muscles
(C1, 2
fibers)

Cover figure:
Cranial Nerves (Motor and Sensory Distribution): Schema

New Terminology and Abbreviations

Summary of the Different Cranial Nerves Using International and Former Nomenclature

I	Olfactory
II	Optic
III	Oculomotor (common oculomotor)
IV	Trochlear (pathetic)
V	Trigeminal, trigeminal ganglia (Gasser ganglia), trigeminal cavity (Meckel's cave)
VI	Abducens (external oculomotor)
VII	Facial
VIIbis	Intermediate (Wrisberg)
VIII	Vestibulocochlear (auditory), internal acoustic meatus (internal auditory canal)
IX	Glossopharyngeal
X	Vagus (pneumogastric)
XI	Accessory (spinal, Willis accessory)
XII	Hypoglossal (greater hypoglossal)

Main Abbreviations Used

2D	Two-dimensional (slice image)
3D	Three-dimensional (volume image)
AEP	Auditory evoked potentials
AVM	Arteriovenous malformation
CT	Computed tomography
CISS	Constructive interference in steady state (inframillimetric slices in T2)
CPA	Cerebellopontine angle
CSF	Cerebrospinal fluid
CVA	Cerebrovascular accident
EG	Echo gradient
ENG	Electronystagmogram
ESG	Electrostagmogram
FLAIR	Fluid-attenuated inversion recovery: T2 sequence with elimination of water
FP	Facial paralysis
IAM	Internal acoustic meatus
MIP	Maximum intensity projection
MRA	Magnetic resonance angiography
MRI	MR image
MS	Multiple sclerosis
NF1	Type 1 neurofibromatosis
NF2	Type 2 neurofibromatosis
NOP	Neuro-ocular plane
PFP	Peripheral facial paralysis
Rho, ρ	Proton density (sequence in)
SCC	Semicircular canal
SE	Spin echo
TOF	Time of flight
TONOP	Transorbital neuro-ocular plane
T1	Weighted sequence in
T2	Weighted sequence in

Clinical Examination of Paralysis of the Cranial Nerves and Principal Etiologies

K. Vahedi and M.-G. Bousser

Despite the tremendous progress made in neurologic imaging, the etiologic diagnosis of disorders of the cranial nerves is difficult. Hence, it is important to perform a meticulous clinical examination to determine whether the lesion is unifocal or multifocal and to search for clues that may help pinpoint where the lesion is situated along the nerve pathway, from its nucleus in the brainstem to its nerve ending.

A cranial nerve is a peripheral nerve that has an essentially intracranial pathway. Only the optic and olfactory nerves are exceptions to this rule because they are an integral part of the central nervous system. Accordingly, the principal disorders of the cranial nerves have diverse etiologies:

- On one hand, there are general causes involved in disorders of the peripheral nerves.
- On the other hand, there are local causes (with disorders of the brainstem, the bony structures of the skull, the orbit, the meninges or subarachnoid spaces, superficial soft tissues).

The clinical assessment of each pair of cranial nerves is described; when compared with the different topographic syndromes, these elements can help the clinician decide whether the lesion is peripheral, intracranial, or extracranial.

CLINICAL ASSESSMENT OF THE CRANIAL NERVES

For the **olfactory nerve** (I), the patient history should indicate whether anosmia or hyposmia is present; this is only the case when involvement is bilateral. Sense of smell is best tested one naris at a time, using well-known odors. The **optic nerve** (II) is assessed by studying the visual acuity of each eye individually using standard scales to determine near and distant vision and by performing an examination of the eye fundus at the bedside using an ophthalmoscope and by studying the visual field.

The III, IV, and VI nerves make up the **oculomotor nerves**. Disorders of the **oculomotor nerve** (III) produce diplopia (vertical, horizontal, or oblique); a fall in the upper eyelid (ptosis); divergent strabismus; reduced adduction, elevation, and lowering of the eye (impairment of the medial rectus, superior rectus, inferior rectus, and inferior oblique muscles); paralytic mydriasis; and paralysis of accommodation. A lesion in the **trochlear nerve** (IV) produces vertical diplopia when the patient looks downward toward the uninvolved side (impairment of the superior oblique muscle). To compensate for diplopia, the patient usually tilts and rotates his or her head toward the affected side. A lesion in the **abducens nerve** (VI) is accompanied by horizontal diplopia, convergent strabismus, and limited abduction of the affected eye due to impaired function of the lateral rectus muscle.

The *trigeminal nerve* (V) is a mixed nerve providing sensory innervation to the face (with the exception of the "notch of the masseter," which is innervated by the C2 nerve) and motor innervation to the masticatory muscles. Clinically, damage to this nerve produces subjective sensitive symptoms (paresthesias or neuralgia) in addition to hypoesthesia or anesthesia of one half of the face accompanied by disappearance of the corneal reflex. The patient's mouth becomes oblique and oval because of impairment of the masticatory muscles, with a deficit in the masseter muscle (i.e., the chin is deviated toward the affected side).

The *facial nerve* (VII) is a mixed nerve formed by a motor root (the largest, or the VII nerve proper) that innervates the platysma muscles of the face and neck, and a sensory root, sensorial and secretory (VII bis or intermediate nerve), that supplies sensitive innervation to the Ramsay-Hunt (geniculate) area (tympanic membrane, posterior wall of the external acoustic meatus, concha of the auricle) and taste sensitivity to the distal two thirds of the tongue. Thus, a lesion occurring in the VII nerve before it divides into its two branches in the parotid gland causes peripheral facial paralysis (impairment of the superior and inferior facial muscles) and geniculate hypesthesia. When the lesion is located before emergence from the chorda tympani, it produces ageusia of the distal two thirds of the tongue. When the lesion occurs before the origin of the superficial greater petrosal nerve, salivary and lacrimal secretions are reduced.

The *vestibulocochlear nerve* (VIII) is formed by the merging of two groups of fibers with different functions: the **cochlear nerve** (audition) and the **vestibular nerve** (equilibrium). A lesion in the cochlear nerve produces tinnitus, hypoacusis, or deafness, whereas disorders of the vestibular nerve are accompanied by a vestibular syndrome (vertigo, impaired equilibrium, nystagmus) that is more intense when the lesion is acute and unilateral.

The *glossopharyngeal* (IX) and *vagus* (X) nerves are mixed nerves that provide motor and sensory innervation to the velopharyngolaryngeal bifurcation. A lesion in the IX or X nerve can produce glossopharyngeal neuralgia (pain in the fossa tonsillaris area). The clinician should look for a tinny voice and paralysis in one half of the soft palate and pharynx (curtain sign). When the disorder is bilateral, swallowing and phonation are severely impaired.

The *accessory nerve* (XI) is purely a motor nerve that innervates the sternocleidomastoid and trapezius muscles and, along with the IX and X nerves, participates in the motor innervation of the velopharyngolaryngeal bifurcation.

The *hypoglosseal nerve* (XII) is also purely a motor nerve that innervates the muscles of the tongue (producing deviation of the tongue from the affected side during protraction) (Table 1.1).

The pupil. The parasympathetic fibers innervating the intrinsic eye muscles and the mucous glands of the head and neck are conducted by the III, VI, IX, and X nerves (Table 1.2). Mydriasis can be the first manifestation of a lesion to the III nerve, occurring before paralysis of the extrinsic eye muscles.

Paralytic myosis from a lesion in the sympathetic nervous system is seen in Horner syndrome, which also includes narrowing of the palpebral fissure and enophthalmia. The long pathway of the sympathetic fibers—extending from the thalamus to the long ciliary nerves, to the branches of the ophthalmic nerve (VI), and passing through the pericarotid sympathetic plexus to end in the short ciliary nerves—explains the numerous possible causes.

ETIOLOGY OF A PERIPHERAL NERVE LESION

Except for the olfactory and optic nerves, the cranial nerves are peripheral nerves. Consequently, any lesion that can cause a peripheral nerve disorder can similarly affect a cranial nerve.

TABLE 1.1 Principal Symptoms and Signs Related to Disorders of the Cranial Nerves

Cranial Nerves	Name of Nerve	Function	Principal Clinical Symptoms and Signs
I	Olfactory nerve	Sensory	Anosmia or hyposmia
II	Optic nerve	Sensory	Reduced unilateral visual acuity; papillary edema; papillary pallor; central or cercocentral scotoma in the visual field (bitemporal hemianopsia if the chiasma is affected, lateral homonymous hemianopsia if the optic bands or the optic radiations are affected [often in a quadrant])
III	Oculomotor nerve	Motor and vegetative	Diplopia (vertical, horizontal or oblique); ptosis; divergent strabismus; limited adduction, elevation and lowering of the eye; paralytic mydriasis; and paralysis of accommodation
IV	Trochlear nerve	Motor	Vertical diplopia when the patient looks downward toward the unaffected side; inclination and rotation of the head toward the opposite side
V	Trigeminal nerve	Mixed	Paresthesia; neuralgia; hypo- or anesthesia of one side of the face; disappearance of the corneal reflex; impairment of the muscles involved in mastication; mouth becomes oval and oblique
VI	Abducens nerve	Motor	Horizontal diplopia; convergent strabismus; reduced eye abduction
VII	Facial nerve	Mixed	Peripheral facial paralysis (superior + inferior facial); hypoesthesia of the geniculate area; ageusia of the distal two thirds of the tongue; reduced salivary and lacrimal secretions
VIII	Vestibulocochlear nerve	Sensory	Tinnitus; hypoacusis or deafness (cochlear nerve); vestibular syndrome (vestibular nerve)
IX	Glossopharyngeal nerve	Mixed	Neuralgia; hypo- or anesthesia of the proximal one third of the tongue and pharynx; ageusia of the proximal one third of the tongue; paralysis of the velo-pharyngo-laryngeal bifurcation; decreased salivary secretions
X	Vagus nerve	Mixed	Hypo- or anesthesia of the pharynx and larynx; paralysis of the velopharyngolaryngeal bifurcation; vegetative signs
XI	Accessory nerve	Motor	Paralysis of the sternocleidomastoid and trapezius muscles
XII	Hypoglossal nerve	Motor	Paralysis of one half of the tongue (deviation of the tongue from the impaired side during protraction)

TABLE 1.2 Principal Parasympathetic Efferents of the Cranial Nerves (Toward the Neck and Head Region)

Cranial Nerve	Nucleus (Brain Stem)	Nerve	Function
III	Accessory oculomotor Edinger-Westphal (peduncle)	Short ciliary nerves	Pupil constriction
VII	Superior salivary (medulla oblongata)	Greater petrosal nerve	Secretion of glands of nasal mucosa, as well as lacrimal, submaxillary, and sublingual glands
	Chorda tympani nerve	Taste (distal two thirds of tongue)	
IX	Inferior salivary (medulla oblongata)	Lesser petrosal nerve	Parotid secretion
X	Vagus (medulla oblongata)	Superior laryngeal and pharyngeal nerves	Mucus secretion of pharynx and larynx

When a single lesion is involved, the lesion can produce mononeuritis and may be part of a general disease process responsible for ischemia of a nerve trunk (e.g., diabetes mellitus, vasculitis, Horton's disease, hypertension) or may be related to a viral disease or so-called essential disorder, without any objective cause (e.g., Bell's palsy). The clinician should look for a systemic disease when faced with isolated paralysis of the III, VI, or VII nerves.

Aphorism: Disorders of the III nerve caused by diabetes mellitus spare the pupil. In effect, diabetes mellitus causes ischemia of the nerve trunk and the central fibers of the III nerve while sparing the pupillary fibers, which are peripheral. In contrast, the pupillary fibers are the first to be involved when an expanding lesion is present. Painful, unilateral mydriasis should suggest an aneurysm of the terminal internal carotid artery.

Multiple lesions can produce polyneuritis (diabetes mellitus, vasculitis) or polyradiculoneuritis (Guillain-Barré syndrome or Miller Fisher syndrome).

ETIOLOGIES OF CRANIAL NERVE DISORDERS IN THE INTRACRANIAL PATHWAY

In the Brainstem

Clinical Presentation

Isolated paralysis of a cranial nerve is only rarely caused by a lesion in the brain stem. A disorder of the long fibers (pyramidal tract, sensory tracts, cerebellar tracts) is almost invariably associated (Tables 1.3 and 1.4).

TABLE 1.3 Principal Topographic Syndromes in Cranial Nerve Disorders of the Base of the Skull

Syndrome	Cranial Nerves Involved	Principal Etiologies
Superior orbital fissure (sphenoid fissure)	III, IV, VI, ophthalmic branch of V, sometimes II (if the lesion is localized to the apex of the orbit)	Invasive tumors of the sphenoid sinus; aneurysms
Lateral wall of the cavernous sinus	III, IV, VI, ophthalmic branch of V, exophthalmos is frequent	Aneurysm in or thrombosis of the cavernous sinus; tumor in the sella turcica and the cranial sinuses
Petrosphenoid bifurcation	II, III, IV, V (neuralgia), VI	Tumors (large) in the middle floor of the skull
Apex of the petrosal bone	V (neuralgia), VI	Otitis with petrositis; petrosal bone tumors
Internal auditory meatus	VII, VIII	Tumors; infectious disease processes
Cerebellopontine cisterna	Sensory V, VII, VIII (cochlear and vestibular)	Acoustic neurinoma; meningioma
Jugular foramen	IX, X, XI	Tumors and aneurysms; carotid dissections
Jugulohypoglossal bifurcation	IX, X, XI, XII	Tumors and aneurysms; carotid dissections
Garcin syndrome	Unilateral, extradural involvement of all of the cranial nerves	Oropharyngeal malignancies; metastasis to the base of the skull

Etiologies

Any disease process that can affect the central nervous system may be responsible for disorders in the intracranial pathway: e.g., malignant or benign tumors, multiple sclerosis, vascular malformations (cavernomas), stroke, inflammatory diseases (sarcoidosis, Whipple disease, Behçet disease), or infectious diseases (abscess, listeriosis).

TABLE 1.4 How to Determine Where Injury to the Cranial Nerves Originates

Brainstem

Isolated paralysis of only one cranial nerve is extremely rare

Injury to the long tracts (tractus pyramidalis, sensory tracts, cerebellar tracts)

Alternate paralysis: homolateral impairment in one or a number of cranial nerves (from lesion to the nucleus or intraaxial fibers) + contralateral impairment of the long tracts (due to pyramidal and sensory decussation)

Cerebral peduncle: III, IV, V

Pons: V, VI, VII, VIII

Myelencephalon: V, IX, X, XI, XII (note that the nuclei of V extend from the cerebral peduncle to C2)

Meninges and Subarachnoid Spaces

Focal or multiple impairment, often bilateral

+/− meningeal syndrome, impairment in other peripheral nerves (polyradiculoneuritis or polyneuropathy)

+/− intracranial hypertension

At the Base of the Skull

According to the location of the lesion in the three anatomic levels of the base of the skull, different unilateral topographic syndromes can be seen relating to one or a number of the cranial nerves, as well as neighboring nervous or vascular structures (see Table 1.3)

After Exiting the Skull

Single lesion (all or part of a nerve): Neuropathies of the chin (numb chin) (V3) and suborbital area (numb cheek) (V2), or a lesion to a dividing branch of VII or XII nerves

Multiple lesions to the cranial nerves: Look for associated locoregional signs (e.g., lesions to the orbit produce exophthalmia plus impairment in the II nerve and the oculomotor nerves in the intraorbital pathway

In the Meninges and Subarachnoid Spaces

Clinical Features. Cranial nerve lesions in the meninges and subarachnoid spaces can be single or multiple. The clinician should look for associated signs: e.g., meningeal syndrome, polyneuropathy, signs suggesting intracranial hypertension (headache, vomiting, papillary edema, uni- or bilateral paralysis of the VI nerve). Cerebrospinal fluid analysis is essential when evaluating paralysis of the cranial nerves, especially when neurologic imaging results are normal.

Etiologies. Cranial nerve disorders involving the meninges and subarachnoid spaces may be related to the following conditions:

- **Meningitis** due to infections, carcinomas, lymphomas, or granulomas
- **Meningeal tumors**
- **Meningoradiculitis and polyradiculoneuritis**
- **Intracranial hypertension (of any cause)**: Isolated uni- or bilateral paralysis of the VI cranial nerve can be seen in intracranial hypertension from any cause and therefore is not useful in localizing the lesion

At the Base of the Skull

Clinical Features. Depending on the localization of the lesion in the three anatomic levels of the base of the skull, different **unilateral** topographic syndromes are seen; these syndromes are associated with impairment to one or a number of the cranial nerves and neighboring nervous or vascular structures.

Table 1.3 reviews the topographic syndromes according to lesion in each level of the base of the skull along with their principal etiologies. The principal difference between the syndrome of the orbital apex and the syndrome of the lateral wall of the cavernous sinus is involvement of the optic nerve in the syndrome of the orbital apex. The association of impairment of the XII nerve in jugular foramen syndrome indicates that the lesion has reached the hypoglossal foramen. Garcin syndrome suggests progressive, unilateral, extradural involvement of all of the cranial nerves by the local and regional extension from an oropharyngeal cancer or metastases to the base of the skull.

Etiologies. These topographic syndromes are mainly due to tumors:

- Bony tumors: Metastasis, sarcoma, plasmocytoma; onset is usually progressive
- Vascular disorders: Arterial (aneurysm, carotid dissection) or venous (cavernous sinus thrombosis); onset is sudden and the clinical course is rapid

Along the Extracranial Pathways (After Exiting the Skull)

Clinical Features. Cranial nerve lesions along the extracranial pathways can be either single or multiple. When a cranial nerve has a single lesion, all or only part of the nerve may be affected. When the cranial nerves have multiple lesions, involvement of the oculomotor and optic nerves in the intraorbital pathways is usually associated with local signs (pain, exophthalmia).

Etiologies. Impairment to a branch of a cranial nerve more often has an extracranial cause than an intracranial cause. Until proven otherwise, neuropathies of the V nerve, chin (numb chin) (V3), and suborbital region (numb cheek) are presumed to be due to malignancies.

CONCLUSION

The diagnosis of cranial nerve disorders is difficult because multiple etiologies can be involved. Close cooperation between the neurologist and the radiologist (and often between the ophthalmologist and the eye, ear, nose, and throat specialist) is mandatory to establish an etiologic diagnosis and to quickly institute appropriate treatment.

Some important points for the neurologist to consider are as follows:

- Determine a precise topographic diagnosis
- Look for additional neurologic and general signs
- Do not neglect the importance of cerebrospinal fluid examination

Some important points for the radiologist to consider are as follows:

- Focus the initial study on nervous structures
- Imaging films should be precise and repeated if necessary
- Do not neglect to perform vascular studies

Cranial Nerves: A Few Important Aphorisms

Intrinsic and extrinsic pain in the III nerve suggests an aneurysm of the terminal internal carotid artery.

A painful Horner sign, either isolated or associated with homolateral involvement of another cranial nerve (III, V, or VII) or a number of cranial nerves (IX, X, XI), suggests carotid dissection.

Until proven otherwise, a unilateral cranial nerve syndrome is presumed to be due to a tumor in the base of the skull.

If the computed axial tomography (CT) scan, MR image (MRI), and cerebrospinal fluid (CSF) results are normal, an angiogram of the brain (conventional or magnetic resonance angiography) is mandatory.

The diagnosis of a syndrome (Tolosa-Hunt, paratrigeminal, Garcin) does not constitute an etiologic diagnosis.

2

Anatomy Atlas

J.-P. Francke

The 12 pairs of cranial nerves are divided into 3 different types (Tables 2.1 and 2.2):

- Sensory nerves: I, II, and VIII
- Motor nerves: III (with a vegetative contingent), IV, VI, XI, and XII
- Mixed nerves that are both sensory and motor: V, VII, IX, and X, with a vegetative contingent in the last three nerves

TABLE 2.1 Review of the Cranial Nerves

Nerve Number	Nerve Function
I	Olfactory nerves and olfactory pathways
II	Optic nerve and optic pathways
III, IV, VI	Motor nerves of the eye
III	Oculomotor nerve
IV	Trochlear nerve
V	Trigeminal nerve
V1	Ophthalmic nerve
V2	Maxillary nerve
V3	Mandibular nerve
VI	Abducens nerve
VII	Facial nerve (intermediofacial nerve)
VIII	Vestibulocochlear nerve
IX	Glossopharyngeal nerve
X	Vagus nerve
XI	Accessory nerve
XII	Hypoglossal nerve

The I and II nerves are not true cranial nerves because, according to their embryology, they are extensions of the primary brain vesicle; these nerves have no nucleus.

The different parts of each nerve are described, but only some of the parts will be illustrated:

- True origin nuclei and intra-axial segment (Fig. 2.1)
- Apparent origin (Fig. 2.2)
- Subarachnoid or cisternal segment (Fig. 2.3)
- Pathway through the base of the skull (Fig. 2.4)
- Extracranial segment

TABLE 2.2 Transcranial Pathways of the Cranial Nerves (Nerves, Orifices, Modalities of Computed Axial Tomographic [CT] Imaging)

Nerves	Orifices	Imaging Modalities
I	Cribriform plate (ethmoid)	Coronal +/− sagittal CT scan
II	Optic canal	Axial + coronal NOP CT scan
III, IV, V1, VI	Superior orbital fissure	Coronal CT scan
V2	Pterogopalatine fissure	Sagittal + coronal CT scan
	Round foramen	Axial + coronal CT scan
	Greater and accessory palatine foramen	Axial CT scan
	Infraorbital canal	Coronal +/− sagittal CT scan
	Incisor canal	Axial CT scan
V3	Oval foramen	Axial + coronal CT scan
V3	Inferior alveolar canal	Panoramic + dental CT scan
V3	Foramen of the chin	Panoramic + dental CT scan
VII, VIII	Internal acoustic meatus	Axial + coronal CT scan
VII	Facial canal	Axial, sagittal, +/− coronal CT scan
VIII	Cochlear canal	Axial CT scan
VII, IX	Pterygoid canal	Coronal and axial CT scan
IX, X, XI	Jugular foramen	Axial oblique (+20°) CT scan
XII	Hypoglossal foramen	Axial + coronal CT scan
XI	Foramen magnum	Axial +/− coronal and sagittal CT scan

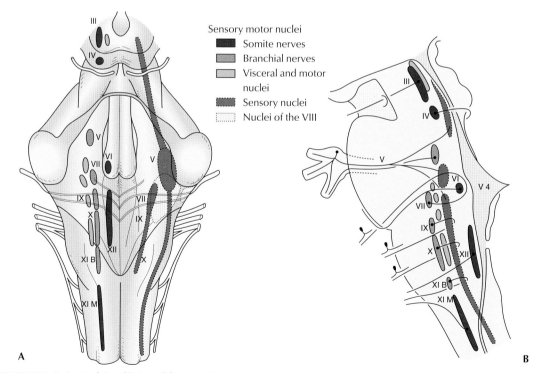

FIGURE 2.1 Nuclei and intra-axial segment.
(A) Projection of the nuclei of the cranial nerves onto the floor of the IVth ventricle (rhomboid fossa). (B) Projection of the nuclei of the cranial nerves and the intra-axial segment onto a sagittal view of the brainstem and the upper cervical spine.

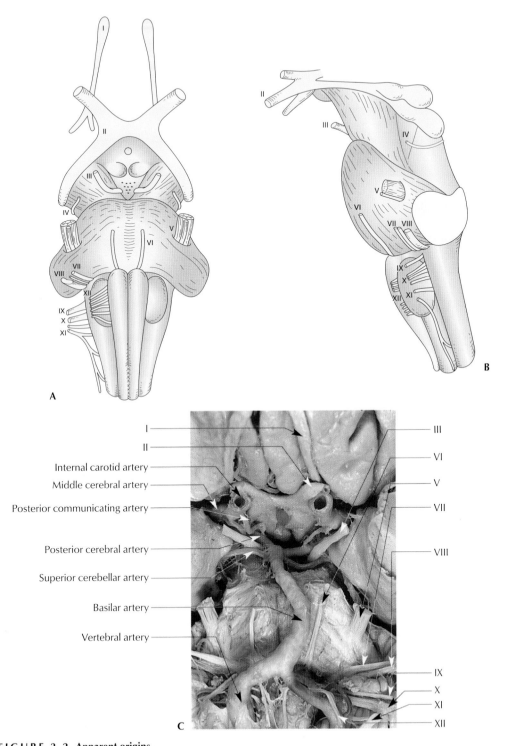

FIGURE 2.2 Apparent origins.
The cranial nerves appear to originate on the ventral and lateral surfaces of the brainstem, except for the trochlear nerve (IV), which emerges from the dorsal surface. **(A)** Ventral view. **(B)** Lateral view. **(C)** Ventral view.

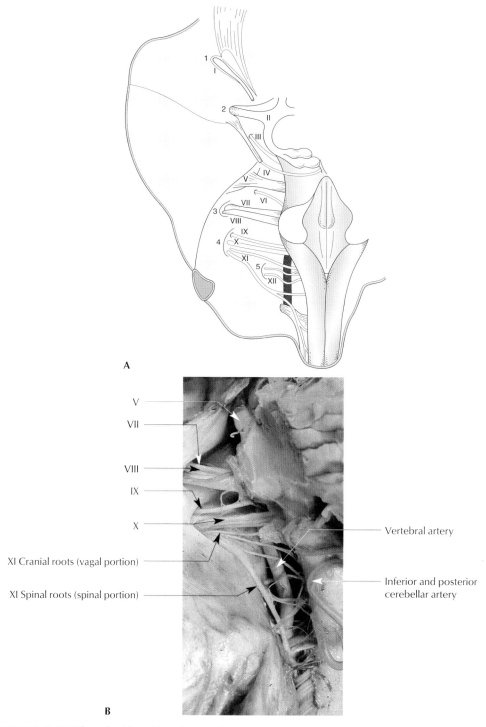

A

B

FIGURE 2.3 Subarachnoid or cisternal segment.
(**A**) Diagram. 1 = Cribriform plate. 2 = Optic canal. 3 = Internal acoustic meatus. 4 = Jugular foramen. 5 = Hypoglossal canal. (**B**) Left posterolateral view after removal of the cerebellum.

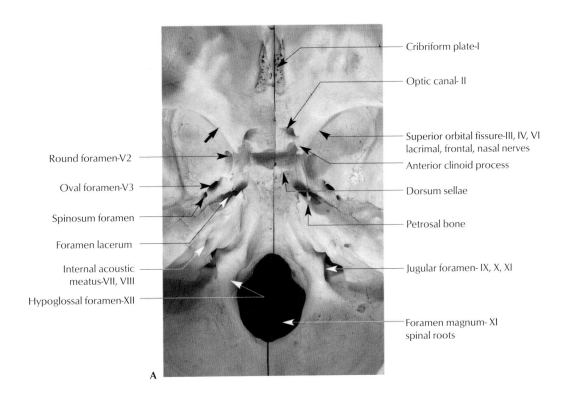

Cribriform plate-I

Optic canal- II

Superior orbital fissure-III, IV, VI
lacrimal, frontal, nasal nerves

Round foramen-V2

Anterior clinoid process

Oval foramen-V3

Dorsum sellae

Spinosum foramen

Petrosal bone

Foramen lacerum

Internal acoustic
meatus-VII, VIII

Hypoglossal foramen-XII

Jugular foramen- IX, X, XI

Foramen magnum- XI
spinal roots

A

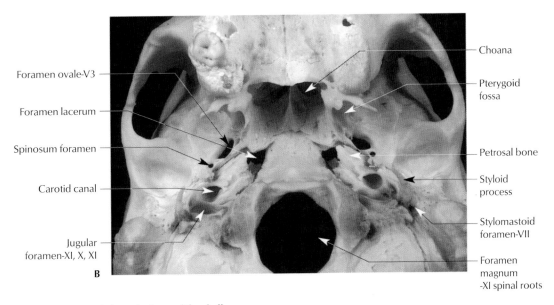

Choana

Foramen ovale-V3

Pterygoid
fossa

Foramen lacerum

Spinosum foramen

Petrosal bone

Carotid canal

Styloid
process

Stylomastoid
foramen-VII

Jugular
foramen-XI, X, XI

Foramen
magnum
-XI spinal roots

B

FIGURE 2.4 Exit from the base of the skull.
(A) Endocranial view. (B) Exocranial view.

- Collateral ramifications
- Terminal branches
- Territory
- Systematization and central connections

CENTRAL PATHWAYS

Central Voluntary Motor Pathways (Descending Pathways)

Voluntary motor function descends along the long fibers after exiting the cerebral cortex (Fig. 2.5):

- Until the long fibers reach the ventral horns of the spinal cord, forming the **corticospinal** or pyramidal tract for the trunk and extremities;
- Or until the long fibers reach the motor nuclei of the cranial nerves, forming the **corticonuclear** tract or geniculate tract.

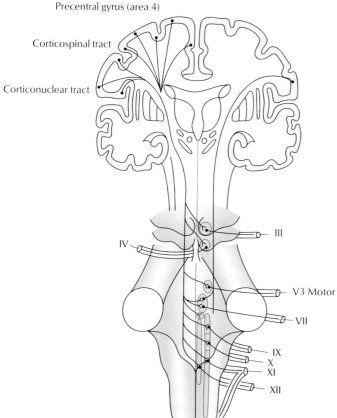

Precentral gyrus (area 4)

Corticospinal tract

Corticonuclear tract

III

IV

V3 Motor

VII

IX
X
XI

XII

FIGURE 2.5 Central motor pathways.

These tracts constitute the crossed bineuronal chains; the geniculate tract crosses over at the different levels of the brainstem. The superior facial nucleus receives fibers from both hemispheres, thus explaining the fact that a central facial nerve lesion does not produce impaired function in the corresponding upper half of the face.

Central Sensory Pathways (Ascending Pathways)

Like the pathways in the rest of the body, the **ascending tract of the cranial nerves VII, IX, and X** consists of three neurons that are crossed. These neurons join the lemniscal and extralemniscal tracts from the spinal cord (Fig. 2.6).

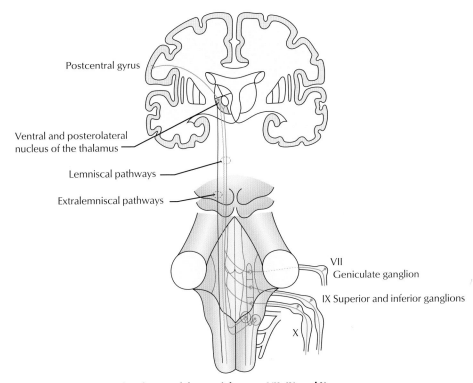

FIGURE 2.6 Sensory central pathways of the cranial nerves VII, IX, and X.

The protoneuron is located in the ganglion, which is appended to the nerve. The cell body of the second-order neuron is located in the sensory nuclei; the second-order neuron joins the posterolateral ventral nucleus of the thalamus. The thalamocortical neuron terminates in the postcentral area (areas 3, 1, and 2).

The **ascending pathways of the V cranial nerve,** which are trigeminothalamocortical (Fig. 2.7), also consist of three neurons:

- Heat and pain sensation in the face and oral cavity are transmitted via the ventral trigeminothalamic tract. The protoneurons are located in the trigeminal neuron (Gasser) and descend via the trigeminal spinal tract to synapse in the trigeminal spinal nucleus. The second-order neurons terminate in the posteromedial nucleus of the contralateral thalamus.

- Fine discrimination and pressure sensations constitute the dorsal trigeminothalamic tract. Their first-order neurons are also located in the trigeminal ganglion and synapse in the

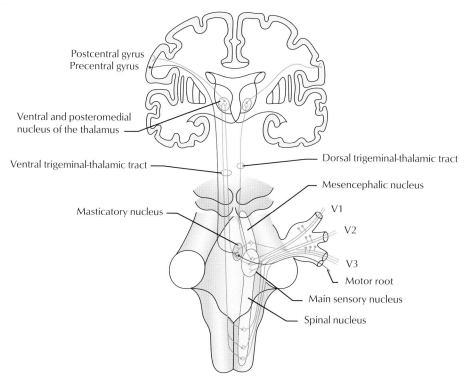

Postcentral gyrus
Precentral gyrus

Ventral and posteromedial
nucleus of the thalamus

Ventral trigeminal-thalamic tract

Masticatory nucleus

Dorsal trigeminal-thalamic tract

Mesencephalic nucleus

V1

V2

V3

Motor root

Main sensory nucleus

Spinal nucleus

FIGURE 2.7 Central pathways of the trigeminal nerve.

principal sensory nucleus of the V nerve. The second-order neurons terminate in posteromedial ventral nucleus of the ipsilateral thalamus.

- The thalamocortical neurons also project onto the somatosensory cortex (postcentral gyrus, areas 3, 2, and 1).

NERVES AND OLFACTORY PATHWAYS (I)

The **olfactory nerves** (Fig. I) are exclusively sensory. They are constituted by the axons of the olfactory cells, or Schultze bipolar cells, which are located in the olfactory mucosa (Fig. 2.8). The olfactory mucosa is found in the posterior portion of the nasal cavity and presents a yellow-pigmented zone and a central sensory zone. The olfactory nerves travel through the foramens of the cribriform plate surrounded by a subarachnoid meningeal sheath, thus explaining cerebrospinal fluid leaks when a fracture of the anterior floor occurs. The olfactory nerves are arranged into two groups, lateral and medial, and join the olfactory bulb, where they synapse with the mitral cells.

The **olfactory bulb** is an evagination of the telencephalon. The olfactory bulb lies in the olfactory groove. It continues into the **olfactory tract,** which is 35 cm long and is located in the olfactory sulcus of the orbital surface of the frontal lobe. Facing the anterior perforated substance, the olfactory tract forms the **olfactory trigone** and divides into the **lateral, medial,** and **intermediate olfactory striae.** The **lateral olfactory stria** joins the lateral olfactory area or the primary olfactory area located at the level of the incus, at the rostral portion of the parahippocampal gyrus. The lateral olfactory stria is connected to the amygdaloid corpus. The **medial olfactory stria** joins

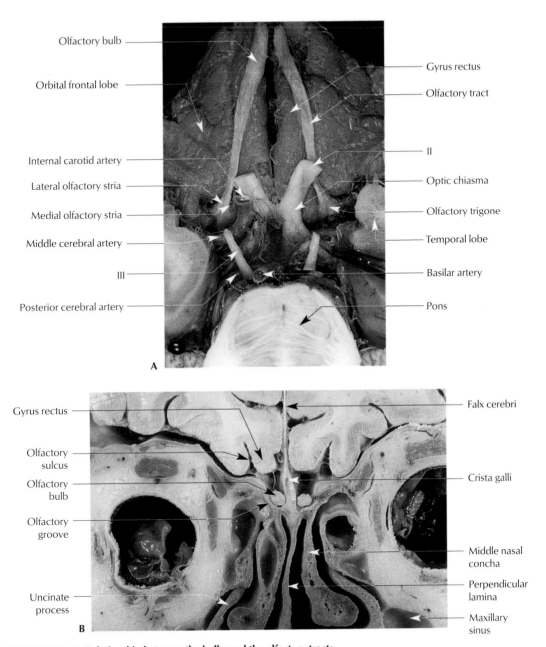

Olfactory bulb

Orbital frontal lobe

Internal carotid artery

Lateral olfactory stria

Medial olfactory stria

Middle cerebral artery

III

Posterior cerebral artery

Gyrus rectus

Olfactory tract

II

Optic chiasma

Olfactory trigone

Temporal lobe

Basilar artery

Pons

A

Gyrus rectus

Olfactory sulcus

Olfactory bulb

Olfactory groove

Uncinate process

Falx cerebri

Crista galli

Middle nasal concha

Perpendicular lamina

Maxillary sinus

B

FIGURE 2.8 Relationship between the bulbs and the olfactory tracts.
(**A**) Anatomic preparation. (**B**) Frontal section of the anterior floor of the base of the skull and the nasal fossae.

the septal area in the subcallosal area below the rostrum of the corpus callosum. The medial olfactory stria is attached to the primary olfactory area by the bandaletta diagonalis.

The **rhinencephalon** denotes the structures of the brain that mainly involve the reception and integration of olfactory influxes (Figs. 2.9 and 2.10).

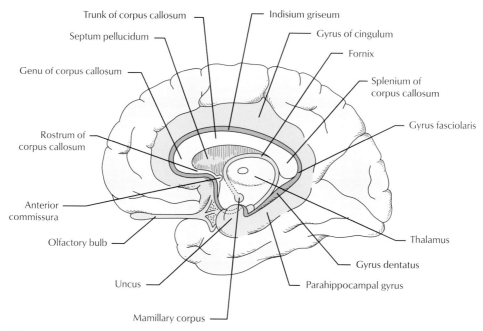

Trunk of corpus callosum

Septum pellucidum

Genu of corpus callosum

Rostrum of
corpus callosum

Anterior
commissura

Olfactory bulb

Uncus

Mamillary corpus

Indisium griseum

Gyrus of cingulum

Fornix

Splenium of
corpus callosum

Gyrus fasciolaris

Thalamus

Gyrus dentatus

Parahippocampal gyrus

FIGURE 2.9 Medial view of the brain, with the rhinencephalon in yellow.

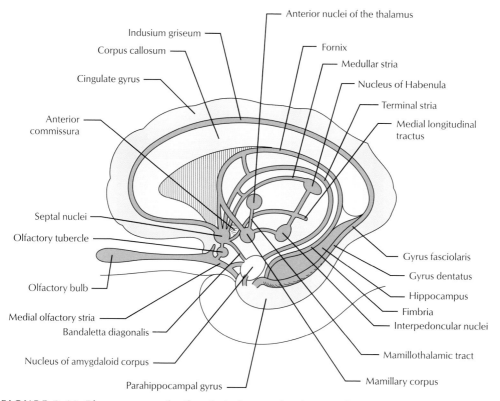

Indusium griseum

Corpus callosum

Cingulate gyrus

Anterior
commissura

Septal nuclei

Olfactory tubercle

Olfactory bulb

Medial olfactory stria

Bandaletta diagonalis

Nucleus of amygdaloid corpus

Parahippocampal gyrus

Anterior nuclei of the thalamus

Fornix

Medullar stria

Nucleus of Habenula

Terminal stria

Medial longitudinal
tractus

Gyrus fasciolaris

Gyrus dentatus

Hippocampus

Fimbria

Interpedoncular nuclei

Mamillothalamic tract

Mamillary corpus

FIGURE 2.10 Diagram representing the principal connections between the structures in the rhinencephalon.

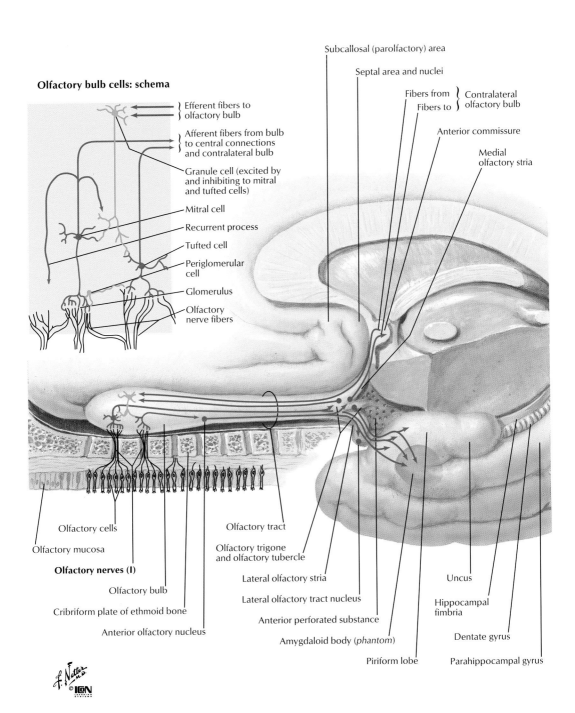

Olfactory bulb cells: schema

Efferent fibers to olfactory bulb

Afferent fibers from bulb to central connections and contralateral bulb

Granule cell (excited by and inhibiting to mitral and tufted cells)

Mitral cell

Recurrent process

Tufted cell

Periglomerular cell

Glomerulus

Olfactory nerve fibers

Subcallosal (parolfactory) area

Septal area and nuclei

Fibers from } Contralateral
Fibers to } olfactory bulb

Anterior commissure

Medial olfactory stria

Olfactory cells

Olfactory mucosa

Olfactory nerves (I)

Olfactory bulb

Cribriform plate of ethmoid bone

Anterior olfactory nucleus

Olfactory tract

Olfactory trigone and olfactory tubercle

Lateral olfactory stria

Lateral olfactory tract nucleus

Anterior perforated substance

Amygdaloid body (*phantom*)

Piriform lobe

Uncus

Hippocampal fimbria

Dentate gyrus

Parahippocampal gyrus

FIGURE I Olfactory nerve (I): Schema

The rhinencephalon contains the following:

- The bulb and the olfactory tracts
- The anterior olfactory nucleus
- The olfactory striae and gyrus
- The olfactory trigone, the anterior perforated substance, the bandaletta diagonalis, the subcallosal area, and the precommissurale septum
- The piriform lobe
- The amygdaloid corpus
- The indisium griseum and the gyrus fasciolaris, the foot of the hippocampus, and the gyrus dentatus
- The fornix
- The stria terminalis
- The cingulate gyrus and the parahippocampal gyrus

Although it is highly developed in certain animals, the rhinencephalon is morphologically and functionally reduced in humans, with certain structures having lost their olfactory capabilities.

NERVES AND OPTIC TRACTS (II)

The **optic nerve (II)** (Figs. II, III), the second pair of the cranial nerves, is composed of all of the axons from the ganglion cells of the retina that terminate at the level of the lateral corpus geniculi, where they relay with the geniculo-occipital neuron (Figs. 2.11 to 2.13). The optic nerve is not a true nerve, but rather an expansion of the central nervous system.

Optic Tracts

The visual system schematically combines the following:

- The **primary optic system,** which contains the sensory optic pathway and the accessory optic system
- The **secondary optic system,** which contains the neuron arc of the pupillary reflex and the arc of the accommodation reflex
- The **tertiary optic system** with the oculomotor pathways
- The **sensory optic pathway** is composed of the following:
- A **reception level:** The retina
- A **transmission level:** Successively the optic nerve, the chiasma, the optic tract, the lateral corpus geniculi, and the optic radiations
- A **perception level:** The primary visual cortex

The **retina** contains two parts that are separated by the ora serrata, the anterior **blind retina,** and the posterior **sensory retina**, extending to the **optic disc** (papilla). It is a proencephalic evagination formed by 10 layers, with the external level 2 levels corresponding to the external expansion of the **cones** and **rods** (layer 4) and layer 9, which is medial to the optic fibers and which joins the optic disc.

The central retina, or **macula lutea,** whose central part forms the fovea centralis, contains approximately 100,000 cones. The peripheral retina, in contrast, contains both rods and cones.

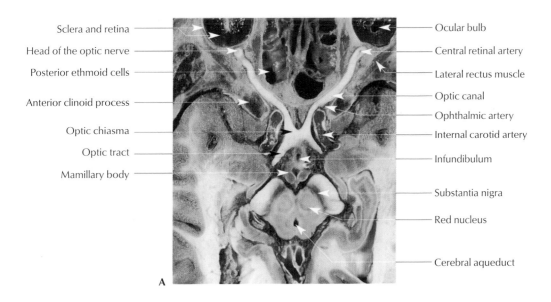

Sclera and retina — Ocular bulb
Head of the optic nerve — Central retinal artery
Posterior ethmoid cells — Lateral rectus muscle
Anterior clinoid process — Optic canal
— Ophthalmic artery
Optic chiasma — Internal carotid artery
Optic tract — Infundibulum
Mamillary body —
— Substantia nigra
— Red nucleus
— Cerebral aqueduct

A

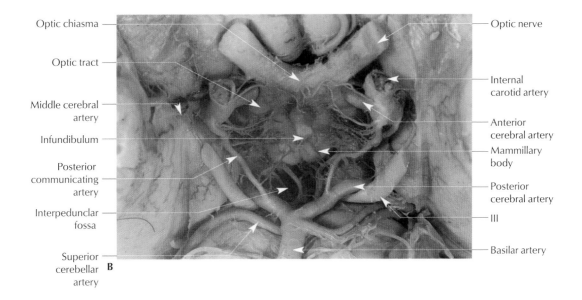

Optic chiasma — Optic nerve
Optic tract —
— Internal
carotid artery
Middle cerebral — Anterior
artery cerebral artery
Infundibulum — Mammillary
body
Posterior — Posterior
communicating cerebral artery
artery — III
Interpedunclar —
fossa
— Basilar artery
Superior —
cerebellar   B
artery

FIGURE 2.11 Relationships between the optic nerves and the optic chiasma.
(A) Axial section near the neuro-ocular plane (NOP). (B) Anatomic preparation of the optopeduncular region and the arterial circle of the brain.

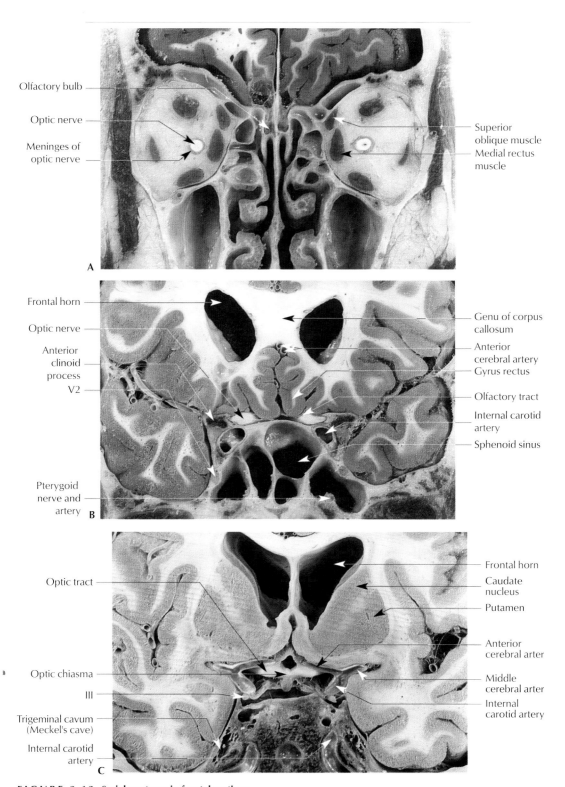

Olfactory bulb

Optic nerve

Meninges of
optic nerve

Superior
oblique muscle

Medial rectus
muscle

A

Frontal horn

Optic nerve

Anterior
clinoid
process

V2

Pterygoid
nerve and
artery   **B**

Genu of corpus
callosum

Anterior
cerebral artery

Gyrus rectus

Olfactory tract

Internal carotid
artery

Sphenoid sinus

Optic tract

Optic chiasma

III

Trigeminal cavum
(Meckel's cave)

Internal carotid
artery   **C**

Frontal horn

Caudate
nucleus

Putamen

Anterior
cerebral arter

Middle
cerebral arter

Internal
carotid artery

FIGURE 2.12 Serial anatomy in frontal sections.
(A) Section through the intraorbital optic nerve. **(B)** Section of the intracranial optic nerve at its exit from the optic canal.
(C) Section at the posterior border of the optic chiasma.   *(continues)*

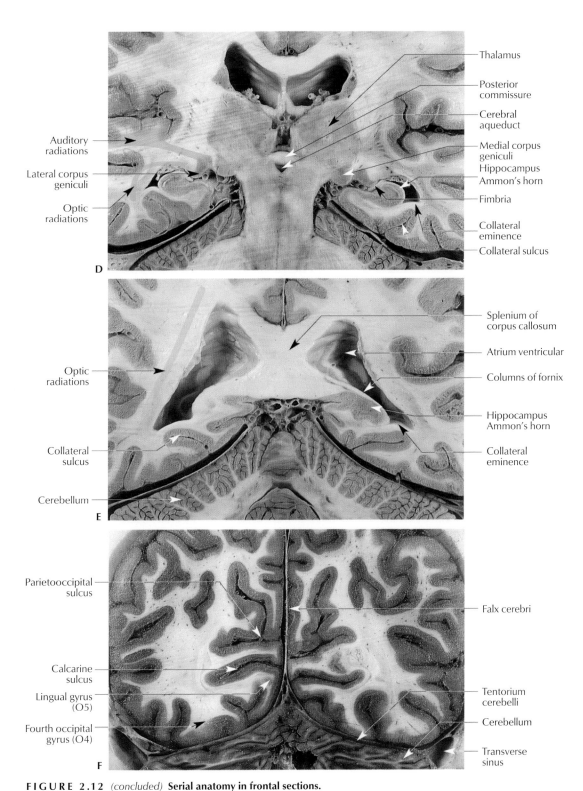

Thalamus

Posterior
commissure

Cerebral
aqueduct

Auditory
radiations

Medial corpus
geniculi
Hippocampus
Ammon's horn

Lateral corpus
geniculi

Optic
radiations

Fimbria

Collateral
eminence

Collateral sulcus

D

Splenium of
corpus callosum

Atrium ventricular

Optic
radiations

Columns of fornix

Hippocampus
Ammon's horn

Collateral
sulcus

Collateral
eminence

Cerebellum

E

Parietooccipital
sulcus

Falx cerebri

Calcarine
sulcus

Lingual gyrus
(O5)

Tentorium
cerebelli

Cerebellum

Fourth occipital
gyrus (O4)

Transverse
sinus

F

FIGURE 2.12 *(concluded)* **Serial anatomy in frontal sections.**
(D) Section at the lateral corpus geniculi. **(E)** Section at the level of the splenium of the corpus callosum. **(F)** Section at the
occipital body.

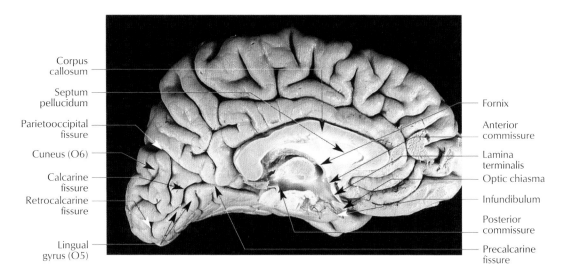

Corpus callosum

Septum pellucidum

Parietooccipital fissure

Cuneus (O6)

Calcarine fissure

Retrocalcarine fissure

Lingual gyrus (O5)

Fornix

Anterior commissure

Lamina terminalis

Optic chiasma

Infundibulum

Posterior commissure

Precalcarine fissure

FIGURE 2.13 Medial view of the cerebral hemisphere and the left occipital lobe.

The optic disc (papilla) is the converging point for the axons of the ganglion cells. The optic disc lacks photoreceptors (blind spot).

The **distribution of the fibers in the optic nerve** is complex:

- In the **retrobulbar region**, the nasal fibers are medial, the macular fibers are lateral, and the temporal fibers are in an intermediate position. In the middle portion of the nerve, classically, the macular fibers move progressively toward the central region, the direct fibers travel laterally (temporal side), and the superior and inferior fields maintain the same topography.

- In the **distal portion of the nerve**, the nerve is oval because of its passage through the optic canal; the direct temporal fibers move toward a dorsolateral position, whereas the crossed nasal fibers assume a medioventral position.

- In the **chiasma,** the macular fibers separate into two contingents, direct and crossed, and radiate like the nasal fiber, whereas the nasal macular fiber effects a slight anterior detour.

- In the **optic tract**, the macular fibers are located in a dorsolateral position. The fibers are twisted, causing the fibers of the two superior retinas to assume a medial position, whereas the fibers of the two inferior retinas become lateral.

As a result

- The retinal field and the optic nerve are divided into two sectors: temporal and nasal
- The nasal fibers decussate at the chiasma
- The homonymous fibers project onto the contralateral hemisphere; consequently, each hemisphere perceives the contralateral visual field
- The macular fibers project bilaterally to the posterior portion of the primary cortex

The **lateral geniculate body** is not just a simple relay; information from the two homonymous hemiretinas is projected, "point by point," onto it.

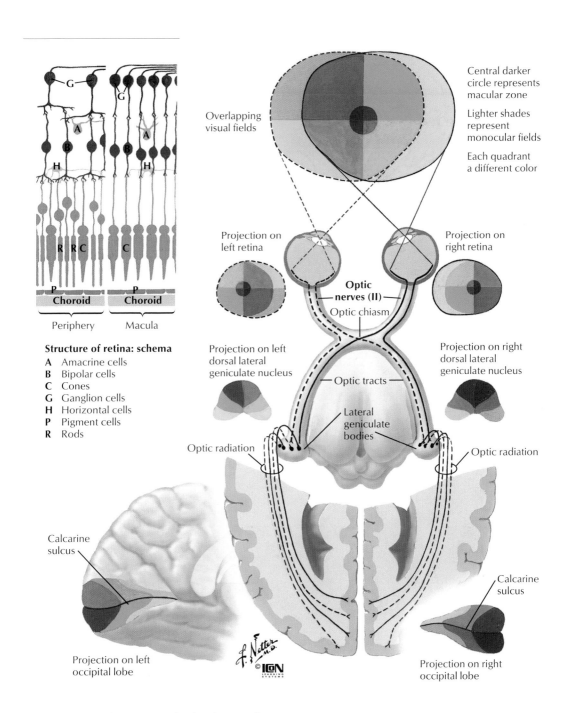

Overlapping visual fields

Central darker circle represents macular zone

Lighter shades represent monocular fields

Each quadrant a different color

Projection on left retina

Projection on right retina

Optic nerves (II)

Optic chiasm

Projection on left dorsal lateral geniculate nucleus

Projection on right dorsal lateral geniculate nucleus

Optic tracts

Lateral geniculate bodies

Optic radiation

Optic radiation

Calcarine sulcus

Calcarine sulcus

Projection on left occipital lobe

Projection on right occipital lobe

Choroid

Choroid

Periphery

Macula

Structure of retina: schema

A Amacrine cells
B Bipolar cells
C Cones
G Ganglion cells
H Horizontal cells
P Pigment cells
R Rods

FIGURE 11 Optic nerve (II) (Visual pathway): Schema

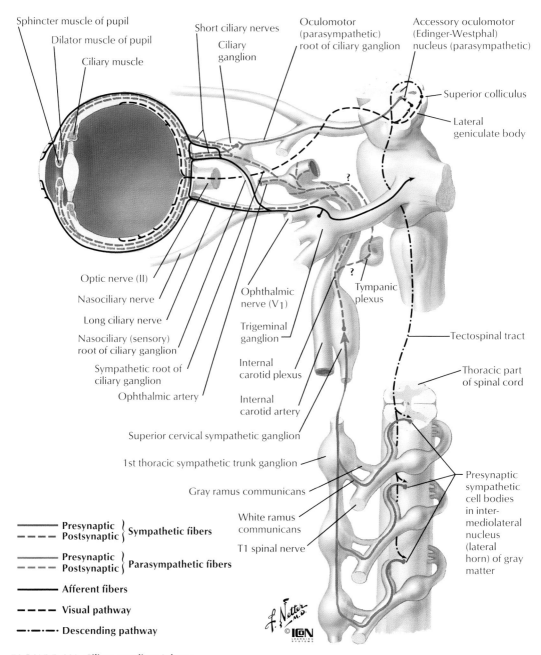

Sphincter muscle of pupil

Dilator muscle of pupil

Ciliary muscle

Short ciliary nerves

Ciliary ganglion

Oculomotor (parasympathetic) root of ciliary ganglion

Accessory oculomotor (Edinger-Westphal) nucleus (parasympathetic)

Superior colliculus

Lateral geniculate body

Optic nerve (II)

Nasociliary nerve

Long ciliary nerve

Nasociliary (sensory) root of ciliary ganglion

Sympathetic root of ciliary ganglion

Ophthalmic artery

Ophthalmic nerve (V₁)

Trigeminal ganglion

Internal carotid plexus

Internal carotid artery

Superior cervical sympathetic ganglion

1st thoracic sympathetic trunk ganglion

Gray ramus communicans

White ramus communicans

T1 spinal nerve

Tympanic plexus

Tectospinal tract

Thoracic part of spinal cord

Presynaptic sympathetic cell bodies in inter-mediolateral nucleus (lateral horn) of gray matter

——— Presynaptic } Sympathetic fibers
- - - Postsynaptic }

——— Presynaptic } Parasympathetic fibers
- - - Postsynaptic }

——— Afferent fibers

- - - Visual pathway

—·—·— Descending pathway

FIGURE III Ciliary ganglion: Schema

The **optic radiations** (Gratiolet radiations) are formed by the axons of the geniculocortical neurons. The geniculocortical tract originates on the dorsolateral surface of the dorsal nucleus, joins the retrolenticular segment of the internal capsule, and slides between internal capsule above it and the roof of the transversal fissure, and finally reaches the anterior horn below. Thus, the geniculocortical tract passes above the tail of the caudal nucleus. At this point, it is compact and forms the **optic peduncle**, then flares out onto the roof of the temporal horn up to the ventricular atrium. The optic radiations follow a characteristic loop in the temporal region formed by fibers from the inferior retinal quadrants.

The **primary visual cortex (Brodmann area 17)** is centered on the calcarine fissure; its superior bank is part of the cuneus (O6) and its inferior bank is part of the medial occipitotemporal gyrus (O5-T5). The primary visual cortex is surrounded by the secondary visual or the visuopsychic perception areas (area 18) and the associative or visuognostic recognition area (area 19). The visual cortex, which has a heterotypic structure, is formed by six layers. Each superior or inferior retinal quadrant respectively projects onto its superior and inferior lips.

Serial frontal sections (Fig. 2.12) from the orbit to the occipital pole offer an overall view of the entire optic tracts and their relationships.

Optic Nerve

The optic nerve contains from 1 to 1.2 million myelinated axons. The optic nerve extends from the papilla to the anterior angle of the chiasma and has three portions:

- An intraorbital portion
- An intracanalar portion
- An intracranial portion

Envelopes

The meninges accompany the optic nerve up to the posterior pole of the mesencephalon. The dura mater envelops the nerve from the endocranial orifice of the optic canal to the sclera. The area situated between the arachnoid and the pia mater is continuous with the intracranial subarachnoid space. The intracranial portion is covered only by the pia mater. The episcleral lamina (or Tenon capsule) extends along the optic nerve.

Vascularization

The arteries come from the ophthalmic artery and the intracranial and intracanalicular portions have only a centripetal peripheral vascularization that is provided by the pial arteries. The anterior segment of the intraorbital portion also receives an axial system that is provided by the **central retinal artery**, which usually comes directly from the ophthalmic or the long medial ciliary artery, or infrequently, from another orbital artery.

Description and Relationships

The optic nerve contains three portions:

- The **intraorbital portion,** which is divided into two segments: the intraocular segment, or retrolaminal portion of the papilla; and the orbital segment, which is 2.5 cm long, 3- to 4-mm in diameter, and forms an obliquely elongated italic S toward the back and medially. The nerve forms the axis of the musculoaponeurotic cone. Through the intermediary of the adipose body of the orbit, the intraorbital portion is proximal to the ophthalmic artery and its branches; the superior and inferior ophthalmic veins; the ciliary ganglion, which adheres to the lateral surface of the optic nerve at a distance of approximately 8 mm from the apex of the orbit; the nasociliary nerve; and the oculomotor nerves (Fig. III).

- The **intracanalar portion** corresponds to the passage of the optic canal, oblique toward the back, medially, and cephalad, and 5 mm long. The nerve is accompanied by the ophthalmic artery on its caudal surface and is wrapped in the meninges, which fasten it to the periosteum of the bony walls. Through the intermediary of the canal, this portion is proximal to the posterior ethmoid labyrinth medially and toward the front—sometimes it is only separated from the posterior ethmoid labyrinth by a thin lamina (the "remote" posterior ethmoid cell or Onodi cell) —the sphenoid sinus medially and toward the back, and the frontal lobe cephalad opposite the sulcus and the olfactory tract.

- The **intracranial portion,** which has a variable length (10 to 20 mm) and angle according to the position of the optic chiasma, thus producing a more or less open optochiasmic window and a more or less difficult approach to the superior and anterior sella turcica and its hypophyseal contents. When the nerve exits the optic canal, it is proximal to the internal carotid artery (segment C3), which slides under the nerve, sometimes lifting it upwards and medially before it reaches the lateral angle of the chiasma.

Optic Chiasma

The optic chiasma is an intersection receiving the optic nerves at its anterior angles and radiating the optic tracts at its posterior angles. Overall, the optic chiasma forms an **X** that is more or less open, elongated, wide, and thick. The variations in the optic chiasma have been well described by Lang. The plane of the chiasma also forms a variable angle with the bicommissural line, which is larger in young infants than in adults. The optic chiasma forms an approximately 7° angle with the Francfort or the Virchow plane. The neuro-ocular plane (NOP) used by Cabanis for studying the optic pathways allows us to follow the pathways successively from the nerve, the chiasma, the optic tract, and finally, the occipital region. The optic chiasma is proximal to the arterial circle of the brain (Willis arterial circle) and its collaterals.

Optic Tract

The optic tracts form two cords that originate at the posterolateral angles of the chiasma and travel around the cerebral peduncles with two segments, a **prepeduncular**, which limits the posterior angle of the chiasma from the optopeduncular region, and a **circumpeduncular**, in the transversal fissure (Bichat fissure). The optic tracts terminate at the posteroexternal portion of the cerebral peduncle in two roots, **lateral** for the **lateral corpus geniculi** and the superior collicular arm, which attaches it to the superior colliculus; and **medial** for the **medial corpus geniculi** and the inferior collicular arm, which is continuous with the inferior colliculus.

MOTOR NERVES OF THE MUSCLES OF THE ORBIT: THE OCULOMOTOR (III), TROCHLEAR (IV), AND ABDUCENS (VI) NERVES

All of the muscles of the orbit are innervated by the oculomotor nerve (III) except the lateral rectus muscle, which is innervated by the abducens nerve (VI), and the superior oblique muscle, which is innervated by the trochlear nerve (IV) (Figs. 2.14 to 2.16).

From their apparent origins to their endings, the motor nerves are composed of four segments:

- Cisternal or subarachnoid (+ a basilar segment for the VI nerve)
- Cavernous
- Superior orbital fissure
- Intraorbital

Oculomotor Nerve

The **oculomotor nerve (III)** (Fig. IV), the third pair of cranial nerves, is the most voluminous. The oculomotor nerve also contains a parasympathetic contingent that enters into the iridoconstrictive and ciliomotor pathways. The fibers of the oculomotor nerve join the ciliary ganglion and then, through the short ciliary nerves, the impulse reaches the pupillary sphincter and ciliary muscles. The contraction of these fibers produces myosis followed by bulging of the cristalline lens due to relaxation of the zonular fibers. The **nuclei** of the oculomotor nerve (principal and accessory oculomotor) (**real origins**) are located in the cerebral peduncle in front of the mesencephalic aqueduct at the level of the superior colliculus (Fig. 2.1). After an anterior **intra-axial or fascicular** trajectory through the mesencephalic tegmentum, the oculomotor nerve emerges (**apparent origin**) at the medial border of the base of the peduncle (Fig. 2.2).

The **cisternal or subarachnoid segment** is composed of three portions, from back to the front:

- The **posterior postclinoid,** where the nerve slides into the arterial claw composed of the superior cerebellar and the posterior cerebral arteries
- The posterior paraclinoid
- The posterior preclinoid

The **cavernous segment** leads the nerve beneath the anterior clinoid process up to the superior orbital fissure.

Already divided into two ramifications, a superior and inferior, the oculomotor nerve travels through the **superior orbital fissure** across the common tendon ring and, in the **fascia-muscular conus,** is distributed to the corresponding muscles:

- Levator palpebrae and rectus superior muscles for the superior ramification
- Medial, inferior and, oblique inferior recti for the inferior ramification

Trochlear Nerve

The **trochlear nerve (IV)**, the fourth cranial nerve pair, is the thinnest and the longest of the motor nerves of the ocular bulb (Fig. 2.1).

The **nucleus** (**real origin**) of the trochlear nerve is located in the cerebral peduncle in front of the cerebral aqueduct at the inferior colliculus, close to the pontomesencephalic junction. The nucleus is caudal to the nuclear complex of the oculomotor nerve (III). Because of the decussation described with the fascicular trajectory, each nucleus innervates the contralateral muscle.

The anterior **intra-axial or fascicular route** of the trochlear nerve is short. Leaving the nucleus, the nerve travels backward and slightly downward, then crosses the midline (decussation of the trochlear nerve), traveling laterally and in back of the cerebral aqueduct. The trochlear nerve emerges (**apparent origin**) (Fig. 2.2) under the inferior colliculus , on both sides of the frenulum of the superior medullary velum at approximately 4 mm by one, two, or a number of threads that join

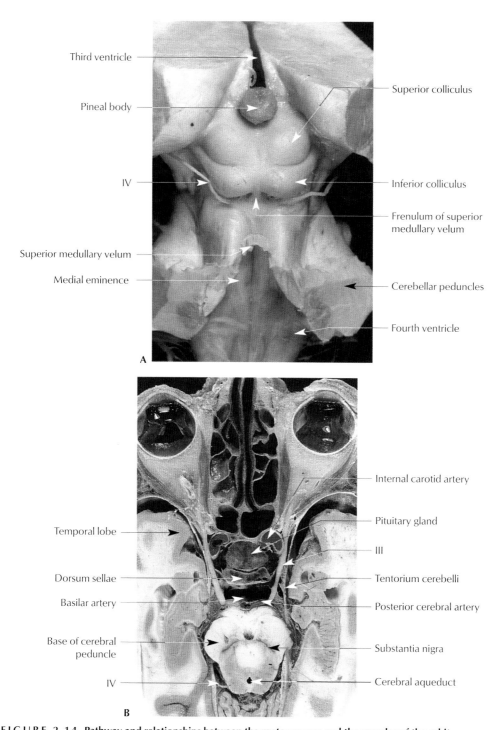

FIGURE 2.14 Pathway and relationships between the motor nerves and the muscles of the orbit.
(A) Apparent origin of the trochlear nerve. Pathways and relationships of the motor nerves of the muscles of the orbit.
(B) Axial section.

(continues)

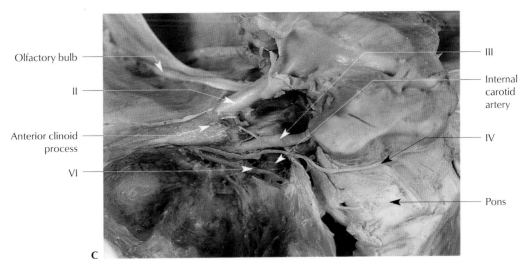

Olfactory bulb

II

Anterior clinoid process

VI

C

III

Internal carotid artery

IV

Pons

FIGURE 2.14 *(concluded)* **Pathway and relationships between the motor nerves and the muscles of the orbit.** (**C**) Lateral view of the pathway of the motor nerves of the eye up to the superior orbital fissure.

together immediately. The trochlear nerve is the only cranial nerve that emerges from the posterior surface of the brainstem.

The Intracisternal or Subarachnoid Segment

Leaving its apparent origin, the trochlear nerve travels laterally between the tegmentum and the cerebellum and appears to be frontal on an axial section. The trochlear nerve passes alongside the tentorial incisure from back to front and below and laterally, crosses the small circumference of the tentorium cerebelli or posterior petroclinoid fold, then reaches and penetrates the cavernous wall at that point.

The Cavernous Segment

The trochlear nerve's penetration is variable at the caudal portion of the dural fold of the free border of the tentorium or at the level of the posterior portion of the pituitary fossa, behind and lateral to the posterior clinoid process and behind and very slightly lateral to the oculomotor nerve. Like the oculomotor nerve, the trochlear nerve is accompanied by a meningeal sheath of variable length.

Further on, the nerves appear to be alongside the external layer of the lateral wall of the pituitary fossa; the curtain of nerves is sometimes separated from the lateral wall by small veins.

At this point, the trochlear nerve joins the III nerve, continues along its caudal border, and slides under the anterior clinoid process. The trochlear nerve is very thin compared with the III nerve. The IV nerve then curves upward and crosses the lateral surface of the III, most often a little in front of its bifurcation.

The Superior Orbital Fissure

The trochlear nerve travels through the superior orbital fissure accompanied by the lacrimal and frontal nerves as well as the ophthalmic veins, outside of the common ring.

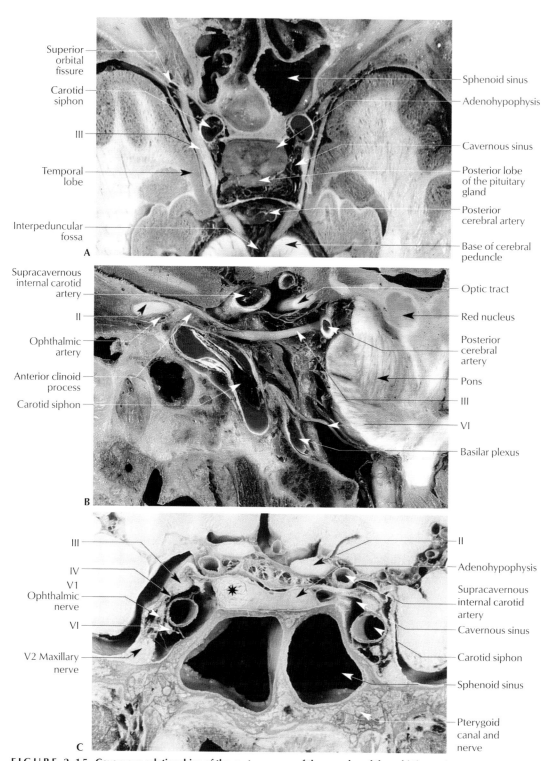

FIGURE 2.15 Cavernous relationships of the motor nerves of the muscles of the orbit in sections.
(**A**) Axial section through the sella turcica. (**B**) Lateral sagittal section through the cavernous space and the carotid siphon.
(**C**) Frontal section through the sella turcica (note the presence of a microadenoma [*] on the right).

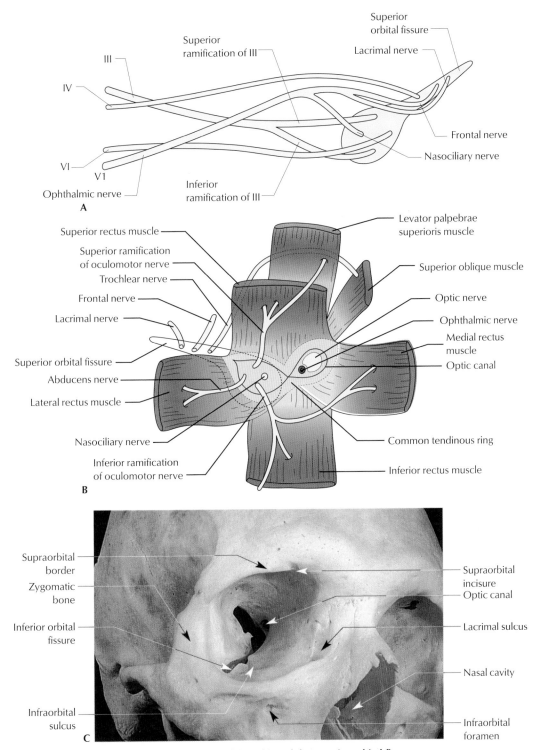

FIGURE 2.16 Motor nerves of the muscles of the orbit and the superior orbital fissure.
(A) Pathway of the nerves in the lateral cavernous wall up to the superior orbital fissure. (B) Diagram of the optic canal and the nerves of the superior orbital fissure and their relationships to the muscles of the orbit. (C) Cavity of the orbit.

In the **orbital cavity,** the trochlear nerve travels along the superior-medial orbital wall up to the superior oblique muscle.

Abducens Nerve

The **abducens nerve (VI),** the sixth cranial nerve pair, is the only nerve innervating the lateral rectus muscle and controls eye abduction (Fig. IV). The caliber of the abducens nerve is intermediary between the trochlear and oculomotor nerves.

The **nucleus** (**real origin**) of the abducens nerve is located beneath the floor of the IVth ventricle, at the caudal portion of the pons, in a paramedian position, opposite the bulge in the colliculus of the facial nerve constituted by the facial nerve's motor fibers, which go around the nucleus of the VI nerve. The abducens nerve contains motor neurons traveling to the lateral rectus muscle and interneurons. These interneurons decussate at the same level to join, by the medial longitudinal tract, the medial rectus muscle III nerve nucleus.

The anterior **intra-axial or fascicular** route of the abducens nerve is oblique toward the front and very slightly caudal and lateral.

The abducens nerve emerges (**apparent origin**) anteriorly, at the level of the sulcus of the bulb and pons, above the pyramid of the bulb, in the form of one or more fascicules that rapidly join (Fig. 2.2).

Five segments are present from the origin of the abducens nerve to its ending:

- Cisternal or subarachnoid
- Basilar
- Cavernous
- Superior orbital fissure outside the common ring
- Intraorbital

The Cisternal or Subarachnoid Segment

From its apparent origin, the abducens nerve travels upward, contacting the anterior surface of the pons. The anterior cerebellar artery crosses in front of the nerve. Next, in the prepontine cistern, the abducens nerve travels obliquely cephalad and toward the front, between the anterior surface of the pons and the basilary sulcus. The nerve then joins and travels through the dura mater of the clivus accompanied by an arachnoid sheath, which is more or less short, as well as a dural sheath.

The Basilar Segment

Further on, the abducens nerve travels between the apex of the petrosal and the dorsum sellae, surrounded by the basilar plexus. This petroclival space is called the Dorello canal. It is limited laterally by the dura mater and the apex of the petrosal, medially by the dura mater of the back of the dorsum sellae, caudate by the petrosphenoid sulcus, and cephalad by the petrosphenoid ligament (Grüber ligament), covered by the posterior petroclinoid fold containing the inferior petrosal sinus.

Most frequently, the VI nerve remains a single filament and passes under the petrosphenoid ligament; however, the nerve is sometimes split in two and one of the trunks slides under the petrosphenoid ligament, whereas the other goes above it. The split in the nerve can be variable in length.

The Cavernous Segment

At this point, the abducens nerve penetrates the posterior pole of the cavernous fossa. The abducens nerve is the most medial of all of the nerves in the pituitary fossa. The nerve maintains contact with segment C5 of the carotid siphon, going around it laterally, and sometimes has the appearance of a ribbon applied to the artery. There, it is slightly ascendant, parallel underneath segment C4 of the internal carotid artery, runs alongside the medial surface of the ophthalmic nerve, then crosses to reach the **superior orbital fissure.** The abducens nerve travels through the common ring along with the two ramifications of the III nerve and the nasociliary nerve. The abducens nerve then reaches the lower surface of the lateral rectus muscle and innervates it.

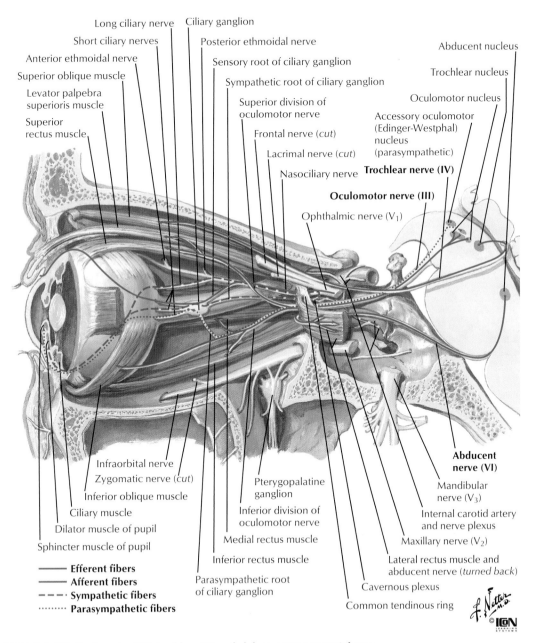

FIGURE IV Oculomotor (III), trochlear (IV) and abducent (VI) nerves: Schema

TRIGEMINAL NERVE (V)

The trigeminal nerve, or fifth cranial nerve pair, is the most voluminous of all of the cranial nerves (Figs. 2.17 to 2.20 and VIII). Part of the first branchial or mandibular arch, the trigeminal nerve is sensorial for the facial regions and motor for the masticatory muscles.

The trigeminal ganglion (**Gasser ganglion**) is found on the pathway of its sensory nerve root.

The trigeminal nerve divides early into three branches: the ophthalmic nerve (V1, **Willis nerve**), the maxillary nerve (V2), and the mandibular nerve (V3).

The sensorial and vegetative fibers come from the facial and glossopharyngeal nerve.

Nuclei, Real Origins, and Central Connections

The trigeminal nerve has three **sensory nuclei** (Figs. 2.1 and 2.2):

- The **pontine nucleus**, for fine tactile sensibility of the face
- The **spinal nucleus,** which descends down to the second cervical myelomere, for pain and heat sensibility of the face
- The **mesencephalic nucleus,** for the proprioceptive sensibility of the masticatory muscles, the temporomandibular joint, the teeth, the facial muscles, and the extrinsic eye muscles

The efferent sensory fibers of the trigeminal nerve, which are mostly crossed, form the trigeminal-thalamic tract and join the medial portion of the posterior ventral nucleus of the thalamus.

The **motor nucleus (masticatory nucleus)** of the trigeminal nerve is located medial to the pontine nucleus, in the branchial motor column, above the motor nucleus of the facial nerve. Its afferent fibers are part of the corticonuclear tract and are mostly crossed.

The **intra-axial or fascicular** pathway of the trigeminal nerve is direct through the pons.

The **apparent origin** of the trigeminal nerve is located on the lateral surface of the pons, at the junction of the middle cerebellar peduncle. The nerve emerges through **two roots**: one that is **lateral,** sensorial, and voluminous (5 mm); and the other, which is **medial** and thin (1 to 2 mm).

Pathway and Segments

Three segments of the trigeminal nerve have been differentiated:

- In the posterior cranial fossa
- At the superior border of the petrosal bone
- In the trigeminal cavum

Cisternal or Subarachnoid Segment in the Posterior Cranial Fossa

The trigeminal nerve travels through the superior portion of the cerebellopontine fornix (cistern of the cerebellopontine angle), whose axis is constituted by the acoustic and facial bundle; and the inferior part, which is limited by the mixed nerves: IX, X, and XI nerves. According to the morphology of the posterior fossa, the nerve can be either almost horizontal or more or less oblique laterally and cephalad.

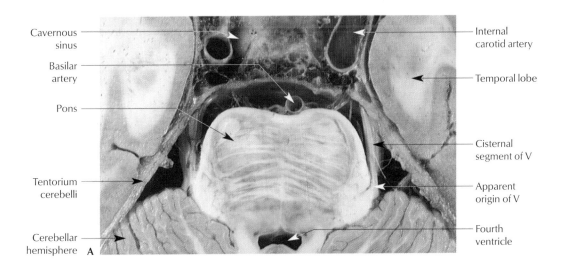

Cavernous sinus

Basilar artery

Pons

Tentorium cerebelli

Cerebellar hemisphere   **A**

Internal carotid artery

Temporal lobe

Cisternal segment of V

Apparent origin of V

Fourth ventricle

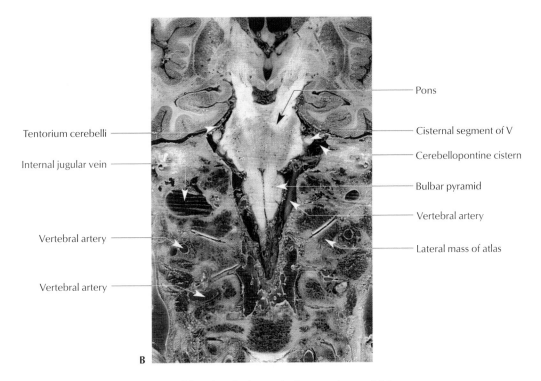

Tentorium cerebelli

Internal jugular vein

Vertebral artery

Vertebral artery

B

Pons

Cisternal segment of V

Cerebellopontine cistern

Bulbar pyramid

Vertebral artery

Lateral mass of atlas

F I G U R E 2 . 1 7 Cisternal segment of the trigeminal nerve in the posterior cranial fossa.
(**A**) Apparent origin and cisternal segment. Axial section. (**B**) Cisternal segment. Frontal section.

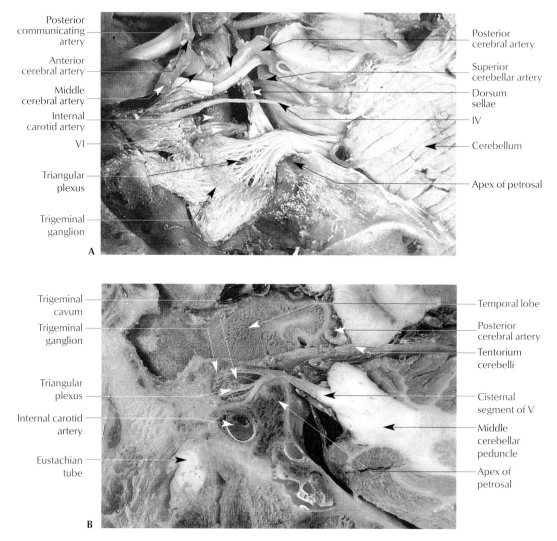

FIGURE 2.18 Relationships of the trigeminal nerve (V) at the superior border of the petrosal bone in the trigeminal cavum and in the laterosellar region.
(A) Left lateral view of the middle cranial fossae after removal of the dura mater and opening the cavernous space.
(B) Sagittal section passing through the trigeminal cavum.   *(continues)*

Medially, at a certain distance, the basilary artery and the abducens nerve travel upwards and a little closer and the trochlear nerve ascends. The trigeminal nerve is rostral to the superior cerebellar artery and ventral to the anterior and inferior cerebellar arteries. These crossovers can produce facial neuralgia if these structures come into contact at the "central myelin–peripheral myelin" junction during the first few millimeters after the apparent origin of the nerve. The afferent veins at the superior petrosal sinus infrequently can also be the cause of the "vein–nerve" conflict.

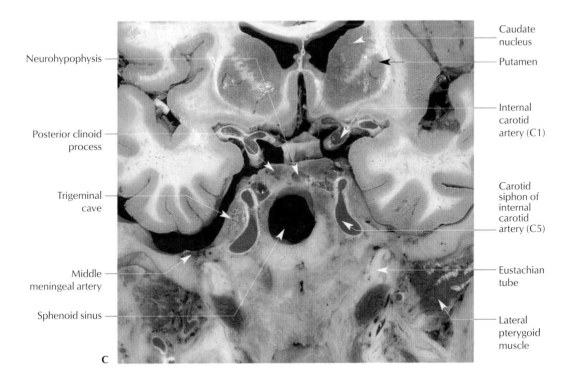

Caudate nucleus

Neurohypophysis

Putamen

Internal carotid artery (C1)

Posterior clinoid process

Trigeminal cave

Carotid siphon of internal carotid artery (C5)

Middle meningeal artery

Eustachian tube

Sphenoid sinus

Lateral pterygoid muscle

C

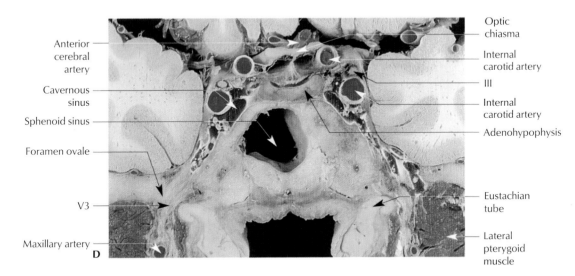

Optic chiasma

Anterior cerebral artery

Internal carotid artery

Cavernous sinus

III

Sphenoid sinus

Internal carotid artery

Foramen ovale

Adenohypophysis

V3

Eustachian tube

Maxillary artery

Lateral pterygoid muscle

D

FIGURE 2.18 *(concluded)* **Relationships of the trigeminal nerve (V) at the superior border of the petrosal bone in the trigeminal cavum and in the laterosellar region.**
(C, D) Relationships of the trigeminal nerve (V) at the superior border of the petrosal bone in the trigeminal cavum and the laterosellar region. **(C)** Frontal section passing through the trigeminal cavum. **(D)** Frontal section passing through the hypophysis and the oval foramen.

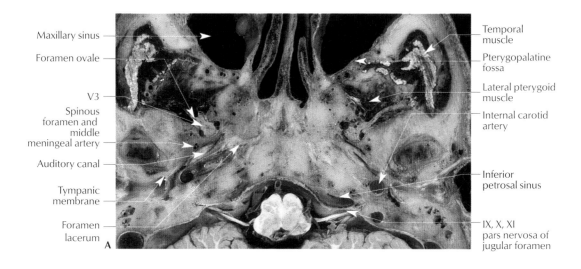

Maxillary sinus

Foramen ovale

V3

Spinous
foramen and
middle
meningeal artery

Auditory canal

Tympanic
membrane

Foramen
lacerum **A**

Temporal
muscle

Pterygopalatine
fossa

Lateral pterygoid
muscle

Internal carotid
artery

Inferior
petrosal sinus

IX, X, XI
pars nervosa of
jugular foramen

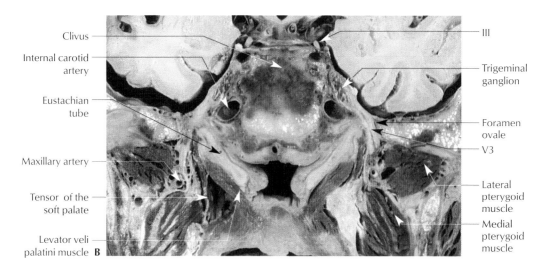

Clivus

Internal carotid
artery

Eustachian
tube

Maxillary artery

Tensor of the
soft palate

Levator veli
palatini muscle **B**

III

Trigeminal
ganglion

Foramen
ovale

V3

Lateral
pterygoid
muscle

Medial
pterygoid
muscle

F I G U R E   2 . 1 9   Mandibular nerve (V3).
(A) Axial section at the base of the brain passing by the oval foramen. **(B)** Frontal section passing by the oval foramen and
the infratemporal fossa.

The sensory root is at first compact and circular; later, it appears dissociated and spreads out
opposite the trigeminal fissure at the superior border of the petrosal bone and the trigeminal fossa
to form the **triangular plexus** and later the **trigeminal ganglion** (Gasser ganglion). The motor root
is initially medial to the sensory root but becomes ventral and then lateral when it joins the lateral
and ventral branch of the trigeminal ganglion, where it assists in forming the mandibular nerve.

At the Superior Border of the Petrosal Bone

The trigeminal nerve slides along the superior border of the petrosal bone opposite the trigeminal incisure (Grüber's incisure), which has been transformed into a canal by the passage of the greater circumference of the tentorium cerebelli, containing the superior petrosal sinus in its layer. Afterwards, the trigeminal nerve penetrates into the trigeminal cavum.

In the Trigeminal Cavum (Meckel cavum)

The triangular plexus and the trigeminal ganglion lie on the depression, or trigeminal fossula, at the anterosuperior surface of the petrosal bone, in a split in the cranial dura mater. At this point, the trigeminal ganglion becomes bean shaped, with a posteromedial hilus that is proximal to the filaments of the triangular plexus and whose convexity gives rise to three terminal branches: the ophthalmic, maxillary, and mandibular nerves.

The trigeminal cavum is composed of an evagination of the dura mater carried along by the nerve and accompanied by a shorter arachnoid sheath (which explains the presence of cerebrospinal fluid), where each sheath keeps its own pial sheath.

Through the intermediary of the cavum, the nerve enters into close relationship ventrally with the greater and lesser petrosal nerves and the horizontal segment of the intrapetrous portion of the internal carotid artery (from which it remains separated by an occasionally deshiscent bony strip), then medially with the vertical segment C5 of the carotid siphon, as well as dorsally and laterally with the temporal lobe.

In the Middle Cranial Fossa

The trigeminal nerve divides into three terminal branches in the middle cranial fossa:

- The **ophthalmic nerve (V1)** travels along the lateral wall of the cavernous space and divided into three branches a little before the superior orbital fissure: the nasociliary nerve, the frontal nerve and the lacrimal nerve.
- The **maxillary nerve (V2)** advances anteriorly toward the round foramen.
- The **mandibular nerve (V3)** goes immediately downward and laterally toward the oval foramen.

The Ophthalmic Nerve (V1)

Destined for the eye, the orbit, and the posterior teguments and anterior portion of the nasal cavity, the ophthalmic nerve is exclusively sensory.

Pathway and Segments

The ophthalmic nerve travels along:

- The **lateral wall** of the cavernous space.
- The **superior orbital fissure:** only the nasociliary nerve goes through the common tendon ring. The frontal and lacrimal nerves join the orbit along with the narrow, lateral portion of the trochlear nerve.
- The ophthalmic nerve radiates only a single **collateral**, the meningeal or tentorial ramification intended for the tentorium cerebelli and the posterior portion of the falx cerebi.

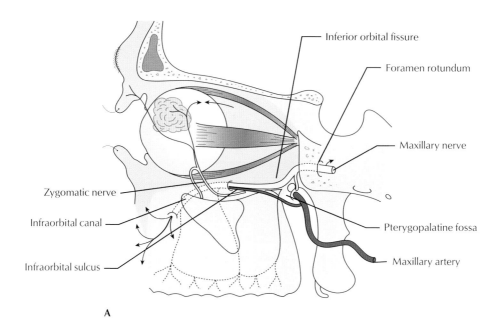

A

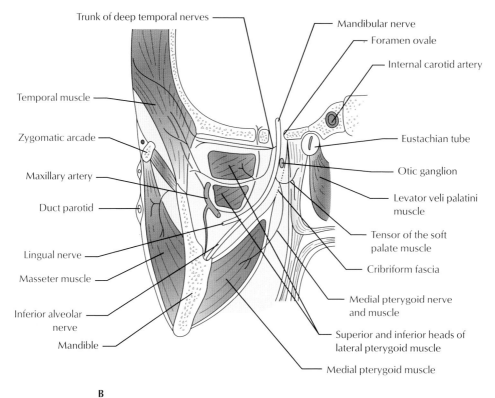

B

FIGURE 2.20 Distribution of the ophthalmic (V1), maxillary (V2) and mandibular nerves (V3), and sensory territories.
(**A**) Pathway and distribution of maxillary nerve. (**B**) Pathway and distribution of mandibular nerve. Frontal section of the infratemporal region passing by the oval foramen.   *(continues)*

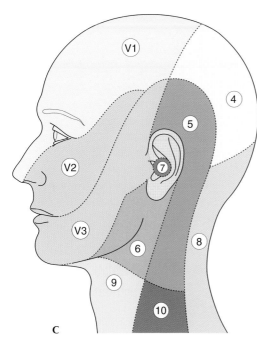

1. V1
2. V2
3. V3
4. Greater occipital nerve
5. Lesser occipital nerve
6. Greater auricular nerve
7. Facial nerve (Ramsay-Hunt area)
8. Dorsal ramifications of C3, C4, C5
9. Transverse nerve of the neck
10. Supraclavicular nerves

Ear = X.

C

FIGURE 2.20 *(concluded)* **Distribution of the ophthalmic (V1), maxillary (V2) and mandibular nerves (V3), and sensory territories.**
(C) Distribution of the ophthalmic (V1), maxillary (V2), and mandibular (V3) nerves and sensory territories of the first cervical roots. **(C)** Sensory territories.

Terminal Branches

There are three terminal branches of the ophthalmic nerve: the nasociliary nerve, the frontal nerve, and the lacrimal nerve.

Nasociliary Nerve. Initially located in the fasciomuscular cone of the inferior surface of the superior rectus muscle, the nasociliary nerve crosses over the optic and ophthalmic nerves from the outside toward the inside; then, accompanied by the ophthalmic nerve, the nasociliary nerve travels toward the medial wall. The nasociliary nerve leaves the cone by sliding between the medial rectus and superior oblique muscles, advancing along its inferior border to reach the internal angle of the eye.

The **collaterals** of the nasociliary nerve are as follows:

- A ramification that communicates with the ciliary ganglion
- The long ciliary nerves
- The posterior ethmoid nerve

The nasociliary nerve divides into two **terminal branches:**

- The **anterior ethmoid nerve,** which travels along the anterior ethmoid canal accompanied by the anterior ethmoid artery, goes through the cribriform plate, and divides into medial and lateral internal nasal ramifications intended for the anterior portion of the nasal cavity and an external ramification (nasolobar nerve) that goes to the teguments of the apex of the nose.

- The **infratrochlear nerve,** which slides under the trochlea of the oblique superior muscle and ends at the medial angle of the orbit in the form of lacrimal and eyelid ramifications intended for the lacrimal sac and the caruncula lacrymalis.

Frontal Nerve. The frontal nerve remains outside the fasciomuscular cone. The frontal nerve travels along the superior surface of the levator palpebrae superioris muscle and divides into two ramifications, the **supratrochlear nerve** and the **supraorbital nerve,** before joining the supraorbital border. The supraorbital nerve also divides into two ramifications, one that is thin and medial and that is intended for the frontal incisure, and another lateral ramification that travels to the incisure or supraorbital foramen. These ramifications innervate the upper eyelid and the frontal region.

Lacrimal Nerve. The lacrimal nerve travels along the lateral wall of the orbit up to the lacrimal gland and passes through it before spreading out over the upper eyelid. The lacrimal nerve receives the communicating ramification of the zygomatic nerve, which brings secretory fibers to the lacrimal gland.

Territory

The lacrimal nerve is exclusively sensory and is composed of the following:

- The teguments of the upper eyelid, the frontal region, the ala, and apex of the nose
- The mucosa of the superior and anterior portion of the nasal cavity and the frontal and sphenoid sinuses,
- The ocular globe (cornea) and part of its annexes (the lacrimal gland, the conjunctiva of the upper eyelid and of the medial portion of the lower eyelid, the initial portion of the lacrimal tracts).

Maxillary Nerve (V2)

The maxillary nerve is exclusively sensory.

Pathway and Segments

The maxillary nerve appears successively:

- In the middle cranial fossa up to the round foramen.
- In the pterygopalatine fossa at the level of its roof, overhanging the pterygopalatine ganglion and the terminal portion of the maxillary artery at the sphenopalatine foramen.
- In the inferior orbital fissure.

The pathway of the maxillary nerve forms the shape of a bayonet sagittally and transversally (Fig. 2.20A) from the round foramen to the orbital floor:

- In the infraorbital sulcus from the orbital floor, where it becomes the infraorbital nerve, accompanied by the infraorbital artery.
- In the infraorbital canal and infraorbital foramen, where it spreads out at the superior portion of the canine fossa. The infaorbital foramen, supraorbital foramen, and the foramen of the chin are lined up along the same vertical line.

Collaterals

The collaterals of the maxillary nerve are as follows:

- The meningeal ramification for the dura mater adjacent to the greater ala of the sphenoid;
- The **zygomatic nerve**, which originates in the round foramen or immediately after leaving the round foramen. The zygomatic nerve remains alongside its root of origin, only leaving the root on entering the orbit, ascending in the periosteum of the lateral wall of the orbit until it is situated opposite the lateral rectus muscle. Here, it radiates the ramification communicating with the lacrimal nerve (secretory ramifications for the lacrimal gland). Then in a small Y-shaped canal in the zygoma bone, the nerve divides into a zygomaticofacial ramification for the teguments of the cheek and a zygomaticotemporal ramification for the teguments of the anterior temporal region.
- The **pterygopalatine nerves,** which travel directly into the pterygopalatine ganglion. Their fibers unite: **posterior-superior-lateral nasal ramifications,** the posterior-inferior nasal ramifications for the mucosa of the posterolateral portion of the nasal cavity and the pharyngeal ostium of the auditory canal; **the posterior-superior-medial ramifications** for the posterosuperior portion of the nasal septum; the **nasopalatine nerve** (or incisor nerve), which also joins the nasal septum by the sphenoid foramen, then travels along the anterior border of the vomer up to and through the incisor canal, and finally divides into the mucosa of the most anterior portion of the palate; the **greater palatine nerve,** which enters the greater palatine canal to reach the anterior portion of the palate; the **lesser palatine nerves,** which go to the posterior portion of the palate; and the **superior-posterior alveolar nerves,** with the middle and anterior forming the dental plexus.

Terminal Branch

The terminal branch is the **infraorbital nerve.** The nerve divides into palpebral ramifications for the upper eyelid, nasal ramifications for the nasal ala, and superior labial ramifications.

Territory

The maxillary nerve is **exclusively sensory** and supplies the following:

- The teguments of the face, lower eyelid and the upper lip,
- The teeth and the upper gums,
- The mucosa of the posterior and inferior portions of the nasal fossa,
- The palate and the soft palate.

Mandibular Nerve (V3)

The mandibular nerve is a mixed nerve, both sensory and motor. The two roots—the **sensory root,** which originates at the lateral portion of the trigeminal ganglion, and the **motor root**—join at the foramen ovale.

Pathway and Segments

In the **foramen ovale,** the mandibular nerve is accompanied by the meningeal artery and especially by the veins draining the cavernous sinus toward the pterygoid plexus. In the **interpterygoid region,** the trunk of the mandibular nerve is very short (<10 mm) and radiates its terminal branches. The **otic ganglion** is located on the medial surface of this nerve.

Collateral

The collateral of the mandibular nerve is the **meningeal ramification.** This collateral originates at the exit of the oval foramen and, along with the middle cerebral artery, joins the dura mater in the middle cranial fossa by the spinous foramen.

Terminal Branches

The terminal branches of the mandibular nerve usually divide into two trunks: the **anterior,** which is mostly motor; and the **posterior,** which is mostly sensory. The lingual and inferior alveolar branches are sometimes considered the terminal branches and the other nerves are described as the collaterals.

Anterior Trunk. The ramifications of the anterior trunk of the mandibular nerve slide over the pterygotemporomandibular fascia. They are constituted by the following:

- The **temporobuccal nerve,** which slides between the two bundles of the lateral pterygoid muscle (lateral pterygoid nerve), then divides into the deep anterior temporal nerve for the deep surface of the temporal muscle and the sensory buccal nerve for the teguments of the cheek region, the mucosa of the cheek, and the posterior portion of the oral vestibule.
- The **deep middle temporal nerve,** which travels to the temporal muscle.
- The **temporomasseter nerve,** which divides into the deep posterior temporal nerve for the temporal muscle and the masseter nerve for the masseter muscle and which travels through the mandibular incisure.

Posterior Trunk. The posterior trunk of the mandibular nerve is constituted by the following:

- The **common trunk** of the nerves of the medial pterygoid, the tensor of the tympanic membrane, and the soft palate tensor muscles that travel through the cribriform fascia (the superior portion of the interpterygoid fascia).
- The **auriculotemporal nerve.** This nerve is sometimes in the form of a plexus at its origin and produces a button-hole for the middle meningeal artery. The auricotemporal nerve travels parallel to the maxillary artery and backwards up to the neck of the condyle, then crosses the superficial temporal artery medially and bends at a right angle to climb behind this artery. The auricotemporal nerve radiates the following: articular ramifications, anterior auricular ramifications, nerve fibers to the external acoustic meatus, a ramification for the tympanic membrane, and parotid ramifications (secretory nerve endings that arrive from the inferior salivary nucleus, an annex of the IX, the tympanic nerve, the tympanic plexus, the deep petrosal nerve, and the otic ganglion).
- The lingual nerve:
  1. In the **interpterygoid region**, the lingual nerve is voluminous and exchanges one or more communicating ramifications with the inferior alveolar nerve and receives a collateral of the facial nerve, the **chorda tympani,** at an acute angle and slides between the lateral ptergoid muscle and the branch of the mandibule.
  2. In the **floor of the oral cavity,** then under the oral mucosa parallel to the gingivolingual sulcus, where it is vulnerable to trauma. The lingual nerve then travels along the styloglossal muscle and the superior portion of the hyoglossal and the genioglossal muscles before arriving at the tip of the tongue. During this submucosal pathway, the nerve follows a curve with an anterior and superior concavity above the

submandibular and sublingual fossa and crosses under the submandibular duct from outside-in, at a certain distance from the curve of the hypoglossal nerve, with which it exchanges a **communicating ramification.**

The **lingual nerve** radiates ramifications for:

A. The isthmus of fauces,

B. The submandibular and sublingual glands (secretory nerve endings that have passed by the chorda tympani and the submandibular and sublingual ganglions),

C. The anterior two thirds of the tongue.

The inferior alveolar nerve:

1. In the **interpterygoid region,** the inferior alveolar nerve separates from the lingual nerve at a right angle. The inferior alveolar nerve is crossed medially by the chorda tympani and laterally by the maxillary artery. Before joining the mandibular foramen, this nerve radiates the **mylohyoid nerve** for the mylohyoid muscle and the anterior belly of the digastric muscle. Anesthesia for the inferior alveolar nerve is performed at the level of the lingula mandibulae.

2. In the **mandibular canal**, the inferior alveolar nerve is accompanied by the inferior alveolar artery. The nerve goes through the mandibular canal, radiating inferior alveolar and gingival ramifications. After having radiated the **incisor nerve** that enters into the incisor canal, the inferior alveolar nerve ends at the level of the foramen of the chin in the **mental nerve**, which divides into **chin and inferior labial ramifications.** With tooth loss and involution of alveolar bor e, the foramen of the chin can be pushed backwards and open into the superior border of the body of the mandible, beneath its mucosa.

Territories

Sensitive. The sensory territory of the mandibular nerve supplies the following:

- The dura mater of the middle cranial fossa,
- The teguments of the temporal region, the tragus and the ear lobe, the parotid-masseter region (except for the angle of the mandibule, which is innervated by the greater auricular nerve of the cervical plexus), the cheek, the lower lip, and the chin,
- The mucosa of the isthmus of fauces, the cheek, the lip, gums, and lower teeth,
- The mucosa of the anterior two thirds of the tongue.

Motor. The motor territory of the mandibular nerve covers the following:

- The masticatory muscles,
- The mylohoid muscle and the anterior belly of the digastric muscle,
- The tensor of the soft palate muscle.

Sensory. The sensory territory of the mandibular nerve includes nerve fibers borrowed from the anterior two thirds of the tongue passed in transit by the lingual nerve, the chorda tympani, and then the facial and intermediate nerves up to the superior gustatory nucleus.

Vegetative. Vegetative territory of the mandibular nerve includes borrowed secretory fibers destined to the salivary glands:

- For the **submandibular** and **sublingual glands:** From the superior salivary nucleus (VII), following the facial nerve, the chorda tympani, and then passing in transit by the lingual nerve.
- For the **parotid gland:** From the inferior salivary nucleus (IX), the glossopharyngeal nerve, the tympanic plexus and nerve, the deep petrosal nerve, the otic ganglion, and the auriculotemporal nerve.

Ganglions

Ciliary Ganglion

Location. The ciliary ganglion is located on the medial surface of the optic nerve.
   Afferents. There are three afferents of the ciliary ganglion:

- The **long "sensory" root,** a collateral of the nasociliary nerve.
- The **short "motor"root,** a collateral of the superior branch of the oculomotor nerve (see the III nerve) that brings the iridoconstrictor fibers from the pupillary nucleus (III). This pathway is activated in the light reflex (constriction of the iris) and the accommodation reflex by the ciliary muscle.
- The **sympathetic root,** which originates in the carotid plexus and brings the influx from the ciliospinal center of the cervical spine and which then passes in transit in the cervical sympathetic funiculus with a relay in the superior cervical ganglion. A lesion in the sympathetic root produces Horner's syndrome, which is characterized by myosis, enophthalmia, vasodilatation of one half of the face, and a fall in the upper eyelid (innervation of the elevator muscle is in part sympathetic).

   Efferents. After traveling through the sclera at the periphery of the optic nerve, the **short ciliary nerves** of the ciliary ganglion join the lateral surface of the ciliary muscle, forming the ciliary plexus, the ramifications of which are intended for the ciliary muscle, the iris, and the cornea.

The Pterygopalatine Ganglion

Location. The pterygopalatine ganglion is located on the medial surface and slightly under the maxillary nerve, in the upper portion of the pterygopalatine fossa, just in front of the anterior orifice of the pterygoid canal, opposite the sphenopalatine foramen.
   Afferents. The pterygopalatine ganglion has three afferents:

- The pterygopalatine ramifications of the maxillary nerve.
- The **vidian nerve,** constituted by the greater petrosal nerve, which brings secretory fibers originating from the lacrimonasal nucleus (VII) and the IXth communicating ramification (a collateral of the tympanic nerve, which is a branch of the glossopharyngeal nerve) and completed by the carotid ramification, a sympathetic root originating in the carotid plexus.
- The **sympathetic root,** originating in the sympathetic plexus surrounding the maxillary artery.

   Efferents. The pterygopalatine ganglion has two efferents:

- The **lacrimal ramifications,** which follow the same pathway as the zygomatic nerve and the ramification that communicates with the lacrimal nerve.
- The nasal mucosa ramifications.

The Otic Ganglion

Location. The otic ganglion is located on the medial surface of the mandibular nerve, immediately beneath the oval foramen.

Afferents. The otic ganglion has three afferents:

- The mandibular ramifications.
- The **deep petrosal nerve** (a collateral of the tympanic nerve, a branch of the glossopharyngeal nerve), which joins the lesser petrosal nerve (a collateral of the facial nerve, originating at the level of the geniculate ganglion).
- The **sympathetic root,** originating in the sympathetic plexus surrounding the middle meningeal artery.

Efferents. The otic ganglion has only one efferent: **parotid ramifications** that follow the same pathway as the auriculotemporal nerve.

The Submandibular and Sublingual Ganglions

Location. The submandibular and sublingual ganglions are respectively appended to the lingual nerve opposite the deep supramylohyoid extension of the submandibular gland and opposite the sublingual gland.

Afferents. The submandibular and sublingual ganglions have two afferents:

- The **lingual ramifications,** formed from secretory fibers that follow the same pathway as the facial nerve, the chorda tympani, and the lingual nerve after leaving the superior salivary nucleus.
- The sympathetic root.

Efferents. The only efferents of the submandibular and sublingual ganglions are the **glandular ramifications**.

FACIAL (VII) AND VESTIBULOCOCHLEAR (VIII) NERVES

Facial Nerve

The facial nerve is the nerve of the second branchial arc (Figs. 2.21 to 2.23). The facial nerve is a mixed nerve: **motor** for the platysma muscles of the face; **sensory** for the external acoustic meatus, the eardrum, and the conqua; **taste sensory** for the anterior two thirds of the tongue through the nervus intermedius; **parasympathetic sensory** for the secretion of the lacrimal, nasal, submandibular, and sublingual glands; and **sympathetic** for the vasomotricity of the tongue and the salivary glands. Thus, the facial nerve is involved in facial gesticulations, taste, salivation, and tear production.

Pathway

After its apparent origin at the lateral portion of the bulbopontine sulcus, the facial nerve travels successively through the middle cranial fossa, the internal acoustic meatus, the petrosal in the facial canal, the stylomastoid foramen, and finally, through the parotid region. In its intracranial and petrosal pathway, the facial nerve is proximal to the vestibulocochlear nerve.

In the **posterior cranial fossa,** the VII and VIII nerves go through the cerebellopontine cistern and form the axis of the cerebellopontine trigone (angle), which is limited by the trigeminal nerve

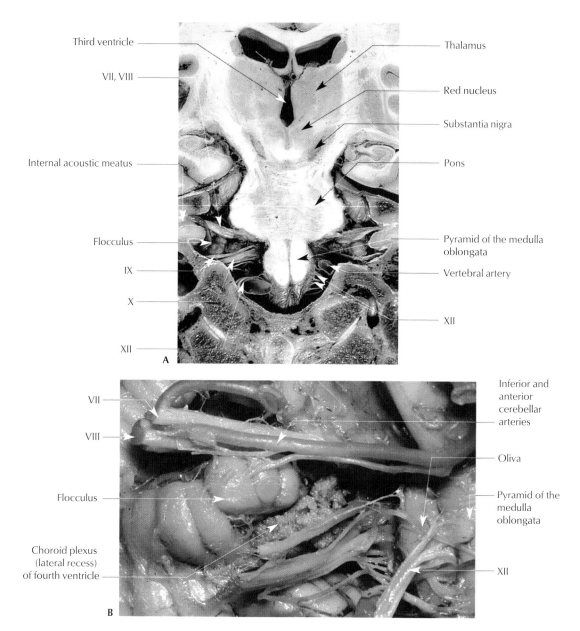

FIGURE 2.21 The facial (VII) and vestibulocochlear (VIII) nerves in the pontocerebellar fornix.
(**A**) Frontal section through the posterior fossae. (**B**) Right ventral view at the cerebellopontine angle.   *(continues)*

rostrally and the IX, X, and XI nerves caudally. The relationships of the VII and VIII nerves to the anterior and inferior cerebellar artery are variable.

In the **internal acoustic meatus,** the nerves are accompanied by the labyrinthine artery, which originates directly from the basilary trunk or indirectly from the anterior and inferior cerebellar arteries (cerebellolabyrinthine artery) cerebellar arteries. The cerebellolabyrinthine artery can

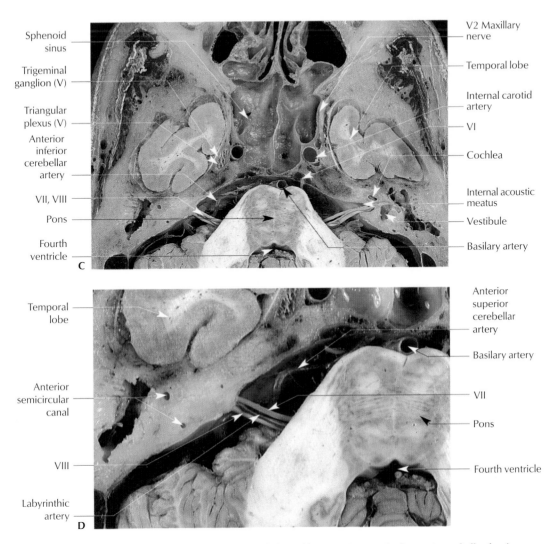

Sphenoid sinus

Trigeminal ganglion (V)

Triangular plexus (V)

Anterior inferior cerebellar artery

VII, VIII

Pons

Fourth ventricle

C

V2 Maxillary nerve

Temporal lobe

Internal carotid artery

VI

Cochlea

Internal acoustic meatus

Vestibule

Basilary artery

Temporal lobe

Anterior semicircular canal

VIII

Labyrinthic artery

D

Anterior superior cerebellar artery

Basilary artery

VII

Pons

Fourth ventricle

FIGURE 2.21 *(concluded)* **The facial (VII) and vestibulocochlear (VIII) nerves in the pontocerebellar fornix.** **(C, D)** The facial (VII) and vestibulocochlear (VIII) nerves in the cerebellopontine fornix. **(C)** Axial section passing through the sphenoid sinus. **(D)** Axial section passing through the left cerebellopontine fornix.

form a tight loop in the meatus. On entering the meatus, the facial nerve lies in the groove formed by the vestibulocochlear nerve, from which it is separated by the nervus intermedius. In the fundus of the meatus, the facial nerve occupies the anterior and superior (facial area) portion, whereas the cochlear nerve is situated below the facial nerve. The superior and inferior portions of the vestibular nerve are located behind and beyond the vestibular ganglion.

In the **petrosal,** the nerve occupies the **facial canal** and is constituted by three parts:

- The **labyrinthine portion,** which is 4 mm long, oblique toward the front and laterally, perpendicular to the axis of the petrosal, and horizontal between the cochlea in front and the vestibule in back. Afterwards, the labyrinthine portion forms an angle of

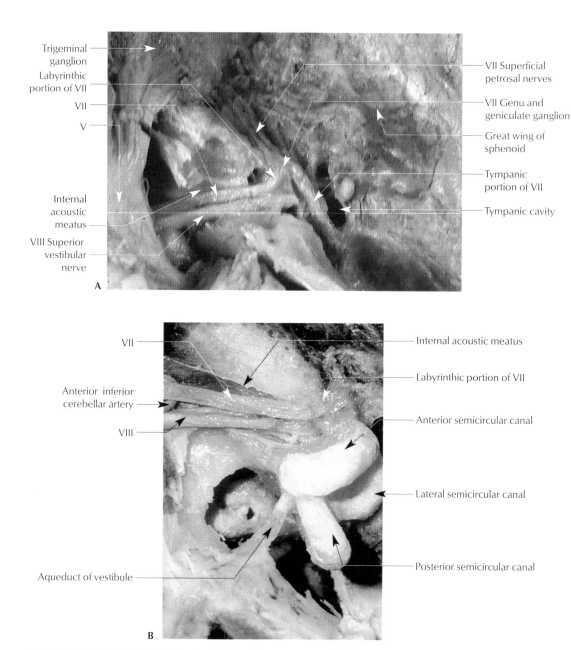

Trigeminal ganglion
Labyrinthic portion of VII
VII
V
Internal acoustic meatus
VIII Superior vestibular nerve

VII Superficial petrosal nerves
VII Genu and geniculate ganglion
Great wing of sphenoid
Tympanic portion of VII
Tympanic cavity

A

VII
Anterior inferior cerebellar artery
VIII
Aqueduct of vestibule

Internal acoustic meatus
Labyrinthic portion of VII
Anterior semicircular canal
Lateral semicircular canal
Posterior semicircular canal

B

FIGURE 2.22 The facial (VII) and vestibulocochlear (VII) nerves in the internal acoustic meatus. *(continues)*
(A) Superior view of the VII and VIII nerves after trepanation of the roof of the internal acoustic meatus and the canal of the facial nerve. **(B)** Superior view after trepanation of the roof of the internal acoustic meatus and the bony labyrinth.

approximately 60 to 70° toward the back, the genu of the facial nerve, where the geniculate ganglion is located and the intermediary nerve ends.

- The **tympanic portion,** which is 10 mm long, oblique toward the back and somewhat laterally, parallel to the axis of the petrosal, below and in front of the lateral semicircular

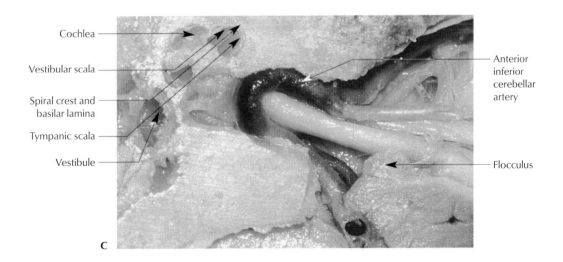

Cochlea

Vestibular scala

Spiral crest and
basilar lamina

Tympanic scala

Vestibule

Anterior
inferior
cerebellar
artery

Flocculus

C

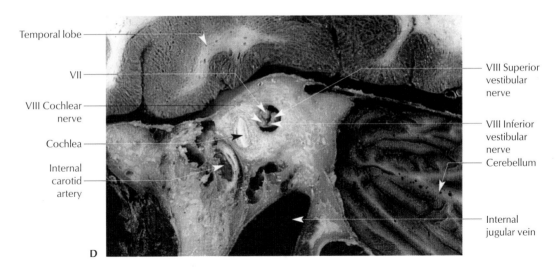

Temporal lobe

VII

VIII Cochlear
nerve

Cochlea

Internal
carotid
artery

VIII Superior
vestibular
nerve

VIII Inferior
vestibular
nerve

Cerebellum

Internal
jugular vein

D

FIGURE 2.22 *(concluded)* **The facial (VII) and vestibulocochlear (VII) nerves in the internal acoustic meatus.**
(C) Loop in the anterior and inferior cerebellar artery. **(D)** Sagittal section passing through the internal acoustic meatus.

canal, under the threshold of the aditus ad antrum, and above the cochleariform process
from the fenestra of the vestibule and the stapes. The tympanic portion ends in the form
of a second angle that is sometimes called the elbow of the facial nerve.

■ The **mastoid portion,** which is 18 mm long, vertical, in front of the mastoid cells, and
lateral and in front of the sigmoid sinus. The facial canal opens into the stylomastoid
foramen, where the stylomastoid artery penetrates, in the upper portion of the
retrostyloid space and behind the styloid process.

In the **parotid fossa,** the nerve enters the triangle formed by the stylohyoid and digastric
muscles. The nerve travels obliquely through the parotid gland, lateral to the external carotid artery
and the venous plane. The nerve then divides in the parotid gland, midway between the tragus and

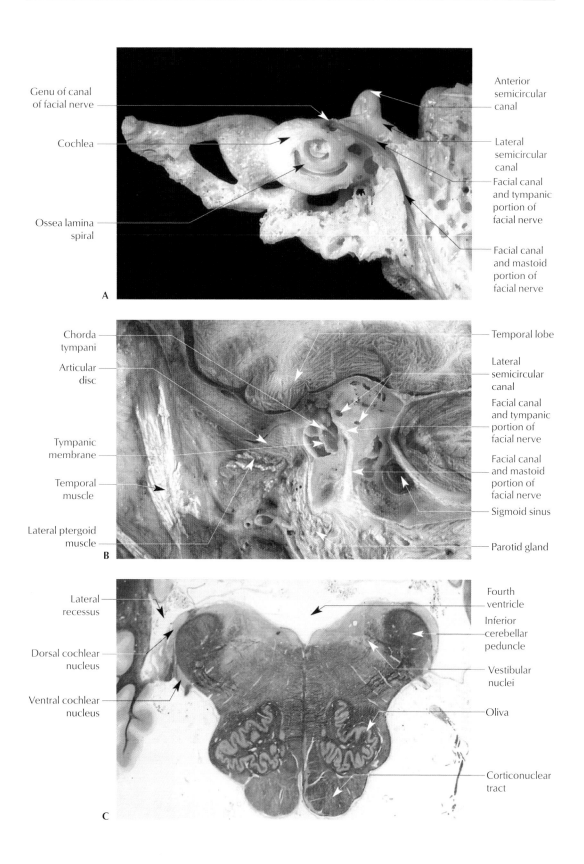

Genu of canal of facial nerve

Cochlea

Ossea lamina spiral

Anterior semicircular canal

Lateral semicircular canal

Facial canal and tympanic portion of facial nerve

Facial canal and mastoid portion of facial nerve

A

Chorda tympani

Articular disc

Tympanic membrane

Temporal muscle

Lateral ptergoid muscle

Temporal lobe

Lateral semicircular canal

Facial canal and tympanic portion of facial nerve

Facial canal and mastoid portion of facial nerve

Sigmoid sinus

Parotid gland

B

Lateral recessus

Dorsal cochlear nucleus

Ventral cochlear nucleus

Fourth ventricle

Inferior cerebellar peduncle

Vestibular nuclei

Oliva

Corticonuclear tract

C

FIGURE 2.23   The facial nerve (VII) in the facial canal (A, B) and the cochlear nuclei (C).
(A) Temporal bone after trepanation showing the cochlea and the facial canal. **(B)** Sagittal section passing through the facial canal. **(C)** Nuclei of the cochlear and vestibular nerves on an axial section of the brainstem.

← *(figure appears on facing page)*

the gonion, into two terminal branches, the **temporofacial** and the **cervicofacial.** The nerve plane and its branches cleave the parotid "like a bookmark in a book" into two parts, a **superficial** and a **deep** part.

Collateral Branches

The **greater petrosal nerve** (superficial greater petrosal nerve), originating at the genu of the facial nerve, travels through the geniculate ganglion, the canal of the greater petrosal nerve, and after passing through the pterygoid canal, joins the pterygopalatine ganglion before supplying the lacrimal and nasal glands. Other collateral branches include the following: The **communicating ramification** (superficial lesser petrosal nerve) along with the **lesser petrosal nerve (IX)** then travels to the tympanic plexus, the **stapedial nerve**, originating on the mastoid portion, travels to the stapedial muscle. The **chorda tympani**, whose origin is variable on the mastoid portion, although often before its terminal portion, travels through the canal of the chorda tympani, then passes through the tympanic cavity by following a curved pathway with an inferior concavity, and finally, through the petrotympanic fissure before joining the lingual nerve (V3), transmitting gustatory sensations from the anterior two thirds of the tongue and motricity to the submandibular and sublingual glands. Other collaterals are the **auricular ramification,** the **posterior auricular nerve,** the **digastric ramification,** the **stylohyoid ramification,** the **communicating ramifications** between with the IX and the X.

Terminal Branches

The facial nerve divides into two terminal branches:

- The **temporofacial branch,** which radiates temporal, zygomatic, and superior buccal ramifications,
- The **cervicofacial branch,** which divides into inferior buccal, marginal mandibular, and cervical ramifications traveling to the platysma muscle.

Vestibulocochlear Nerve

The vestibulocochlear nerve is a sensory nerve composed of two parts, the **vestibular nerve,** which is implicated in balance, and the **cochlear nerve,** which gathers auditory sensations. The vestibulocochlear nerve is entirely intracranial, from its receptors (situated in the inner ear) to the **vestibular and cochlear nuclei,** which are projected facing the vestibular area of the rhomboid fossa, in proximal to the lateral recess. Along their pathway, these nuclei present the **vestibular ganglion** (Scarpa ganglion) and the **spiral ganglion of cochleae** (ganglion of Corti).

Pathway

After its apparent origin at the lateral portion of the bulbopontine sulcus, behind the facial nerve, the vestibulocochlear nerve joins the facial nerve before using the same pathway (see above) up to the internal acoustic meatus.

The **vestibular nerve** transmits information gathered by the **vestibular cells**, which are ciliated cells in contact with the endolymph located at the level of the **acoustic macules** of the utricle and the sacculus as well as the **ampullary cristae** of the semicircular canals. At the level of the vestibular ganglion, the vestibular nerve is formed by the merging of the **superior vestibular nerve** (merger of the **utriculoampullary nerve** and the **superior saccular nerve** or anastomosis) and the **inferior vestibular nerve** (merger of the **saccular nerve** and the **posterior ampullary nerve).** The fibers of the vestibular nerve join the vestibular nuclei of the brainstem, the ampullary fibers end in the four nuclei, the saccular fibers end in the inferior vestibular nucleus, and the utricular fibers end in the inferior and medial nuclei. The **vestibular tracts** constitute a complex, essentially reflex system that is part of the apparatus designed to control unconscious equilibrium related to the archeocerebellum. The vestibular nerve is also involved in direct conscious equilibrium toward the cerebral cortex after relay through the striate body or, indirectly, through the cerebellum before traveling to the red nucleus and the thalamus.

The **cochlear nerve** transmits information gathered by the **internal** and **external ciliated cells of the organum spirale** (Corti spiral organ of Corti) brought by the **basal lamina.** The cochlear dendrites join the spiral canal of the modiolus (columella), which houses the **spiral ganglion.** Afterward, the axons of the spiral ganglion are contained in the longitudinal canals of the modiolus, exit by the cochlear area, and join in the fundus of the acoustic meatus to form the cochlear nerve. The fibers join the dorsal and ventral cochlear nuclei in the brainstem, where the ventral cochlear nucleus has a precise topographic organization. The **cochlear tracts** are thus formed by the deutoneurons that decussate and join the medial geniculate body. These deutoneurons make up the **lateral lemniscus**. Along the pathway, the relay centres follow one another: the nucleus of the trapezoid body, the superior oliva, and finally, the inferior colliculus. The **medial geniculate body** also has a topographic **organization** and projects onto the **transversal temporal gyrus** (Heschl area 41) by the auditory radiations.

GLOSSOPHARYNGEAL NERVE (IX), VAGUS NERVE (X), AND ACCESSORY NERVE (XI)

The glossopharyngeal (IX), vagus (X), and accessory (XI) nerves have a common initial pathway (Fig. VIII):

- **Apparent origin** in the dorsolateral sulcus of the bulb (Fig. 2.24)
- **Cisternal segment in the posterior fossa,** at the inferior portion of the cerebellopontine fornix (Fig. 2.25)
- **Base of the skull:** the anterior portion "pars nervosa" of the jugular foramen with the inferior petrosal sinus (Fig. 2.26)
- **Extracranial segment:** the retrostyloid region with the internal jugular vein, the internal carotid artery, the XII nerve, the sympathetic trunk, and the superior cervical ganglion (Fig. 2.27)

Glossopharyngeal Nerve (IX)

The glossopharyngeal nerve is the nerve of the third branchial arch that contains the afferent fibers of the proximal third of the tongue and the pharynx along with efferent fibers for the stylopharyngeal muscle and the parotid gland.

On exiting the jugular foramen, the glossopharyngeal nerve presents the **superior and inferior ganglions**. Next, the nerve winds around the stylopharyngeal muscle, passes along its lateral surface, slides medial to the hypoglossal and styloglossal muscles, and finally travels between the superior and middle constrictor muscles before reaching the tongue.

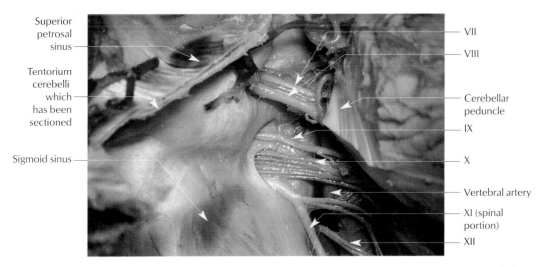

FIGURE 2.24 Posterolateral view of the pontocerebellar fornix cistern after section of the tentorium cerebelli and exeresis of the cerebellum.

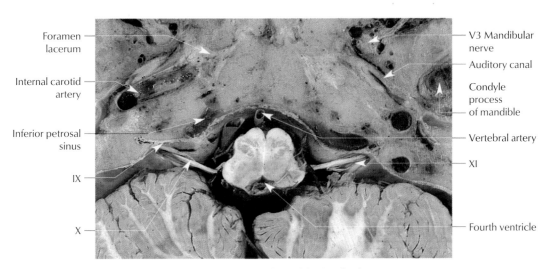

FIGURE 2.25 Axial section immediately below the plane of the jugular foramen.

Collateral Branches

The collateral branches of the glossopharyngeal nerve are the **tympanic nerve,** which radiates, in the tympanic cavity, the **tympanic plexus** and the **lesser petrosal nerve** (for the otic ganglion and the parotid gland); the **carotid sinus nerve, pharyngeal and tonsillar ramifications;** and finally, the **nerve for the stylopharyngeal muscle.**

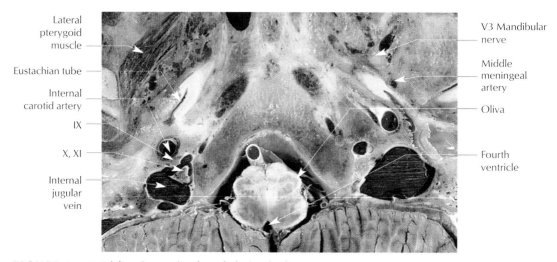

Lateral pterygoid muscle

Eustachian tube

Internal carotid artery

IX

X, XI

Internal jugular vein

V3 Mandibular nerve

Middle meningeal artery

Oliva

Fourth ventricle

FIGURE 2.26 Axial section passing through the jugular foramen.

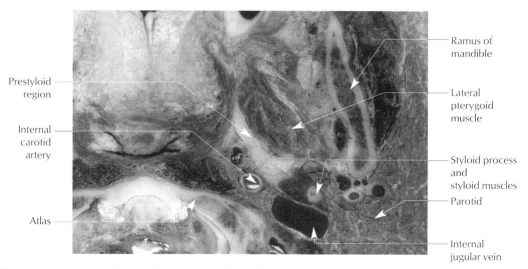

Prestyloid region

Internal carotid artery

Atlas

Ramus of mandible

Lateral pterygoid muscle

Styloid process and styloid muscles

Parotid

Internal jugular vein

FIGURE 2.27 Axial section passing through the lateral pharyngeal space.

Terminal Branches

The terminal branches of the glossopharyngeal nerve are lingual and receive gustatory and sensory fibers from the proximal third of the tongue and the vallate papillae.

Vagus Nerve (X)

The vagus nerve is a mixed somatic and visceral nerve that covers an extensive territory, from the thorax to the abdomen (Figs. V and VIII). The vagus nerve transports afferent and efferent fibers from the larynx and pharynx.

The vagus nerve presents the superior ganglion (jugular) at the jugular foramen and the inferior ganglion (plexiform) in the retrostyloid space. Afterwards, the vagus nerve receives the internal branch of the accessory nerve (XI).

Pathway

The vagus nerve descends in the carotid sheath, in the posterior angle of the internal jugular vein and the internal carotid artery, followed by the common carotid artery. The vagus nerve travels successively through the retrostyloid space, the carotid trigone, and the laterotracheal and esophageal region, where it becomes proximal to the lateral lobe of the thyroid gland before entering the upper opening of the thorax. In the upper mediastinum, the right vagus nerve slides along the lateral surface of the trachea, then goes behind the right main bronchus, whereas the left vagus nerve passes between the left common carotid artery and the thoracic portion of the subclavian artery and travels along the aortic arch and the posterior side of the left main bronchus. In the posterior mediastinum, the vagus nerves form the esophageal plexus, which reconstructs into two trunks, a **posterior** (formed mainly by fibers from the right vagus) and an **anterior** (formed mainly by fibers from the left vagus) in the esophageal hiatus of the diaphragm.

Ending

The posterior trunk of the vagus nerve joins to the plexus celiacus and radiates gastric and hepatic ramifications.

Collateral Branches

The collateral branches include the **meningeal ramification**; the **auricular ramification,** originating in the superior ganglion; the **pharyngeal ramifications** that, with the ramifications from the cervical sympathetic trunk and the IX nerve, constitute the **pharyngeal plexus;** the **carotid sinus nerve,** which joins to the sympathetic ramifications and the ramifications of the IX nerve; the carotid glomus; the **cardiac nerves;** the **superior laryngeal nerve;** and the **recurrent laryngeal nerve**. The **superior laryngeal nerve** divides into two ramifications, a **medial ramification** that is sensory for the upper floor of the laryngeal mucosa, and a **mixed, lateral ramification** that is motor for the cricothyroid muscle. The **recurrent laryngeal nerve** innervates all of the other muscles of the larynx and, in addition, is sensory for the laryngeal mucosa underlying the vocal cords. The **right recurrent, laryngeal nerve** originates from the vagus nerve at the level of the subclavian artery; the **left recurrent laryngeal nerve** originates in the thorax at the level of the aortic arch and travels behind it near the insertion of the arterial ligamentum.

Accessory or Spinal Nerve (XI)

The accessory nerve is formed from the union of a **spinal root,** which originates at the lateral side of the cervical spine before it enters the foramen magnum, and a **cranial root** (Fig. VI). These roots join near the jugular foramen before separating once again into two ramifications. The **medial ramification**, formed by fibers from the cranial root, join the vagus nerve to supply the muscles of the larynx. The **medial root** supplies the trapezius and sternocleidomastoid muscles, thus allowing rotation of the head; it anastomoses with C2, C3, and C4.

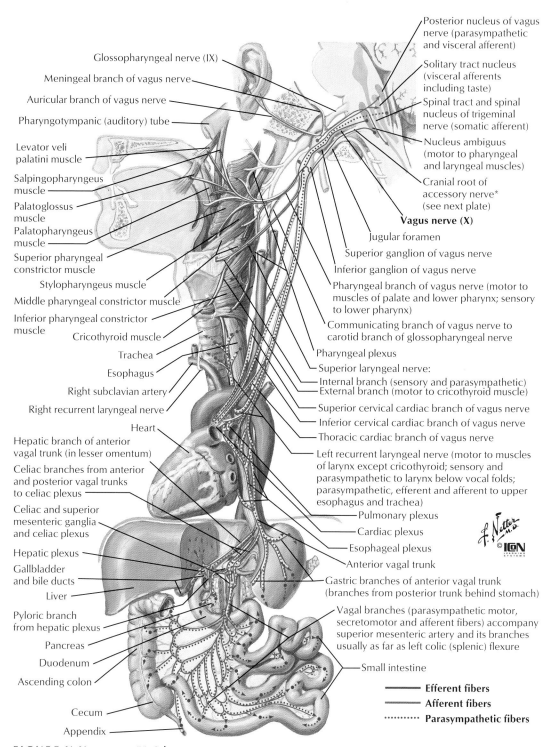

Glossopharyngeal nerve (IX)

Meningeal branch of vagus nerve

Auricular branch of vagus nerve

Pharyngotympanic (auditory) tube

Levator veli palatini muscle

Salpingopharyngeus muscle

Palatoglossus muscle

Palatopharyngeus muscle

Superior pharyngeal constrictor muscle

Stylopharyngeus muscle

Middle pharyngeal constrictor muscle

Inferior pharyngeal constrictor muscle

Cricothyroid muscle

Trachea

Esophagus

Right subclavian artery

Right recurrent laryngeal nerve

Heart

Hepatic branch of anterior vagal trunk (in lesser omentum)

Celiac branches from anterior and posterior vagal trunks to celiac plexus

Celiac and superior mesenteric ganglia and celiac plexus

Hepatic plexus

Gallbladder and bile ducts

Liver

Pyloric branch from hepatic plexus

Pancreas

Duodenum

Ascending colon

Cecum

Appendix

Posterior nucleus of vagus nerve (parasympathetic and visceral afferent)

Solitary tract nucleus (visceral afferents including taste)

Spinal tract and spinal nucleus of trigeminal nerve (somatic afferent)

Nucleus ambiguus (motor to pharyngeal and laryngeal muscles)

Cranial root of accessory nerve* (see next plate)

Vagus nerve (X)

Jugular foramen

Superior ganglion of vagus nerve

Inferior ganglion of vagus nerve

Pharyngeal branch of vagus nerve (motor to muscles of palate and lower pharynx; sensory to lower pharynx)

Communicating branch of vagus nerve to carotid branch of glossopharyngeal nerve

Pharyngeal plexus

Superior laryngeal nerve:
Internal branch (sensory and parasympathetic)
External branch (motor to cricothyroid muscle)

Superior cervical cardiac branch of vagus nerve

Inferior cervical cardiac branch of vagus nerve

Thoracic cardiac branch of vagus nerve

Left recurrent laryngeal nerve (motor to muscles of larynx except cricothyroid; sensory and parasympathetic to larynx below vocal folds; parasympathetic, efferent and afferent to upper esophagus and trachea)

Pulmonary plexus

Cardiac plexus

Esophageal plexus

Anterior vagal trunk

Gastric branches of anterior vagal trunk (branches from posterior trunk behind stomach)

Vagal branches (parasympathetic motor, secretomotor and afferent fibers) accompany superior mesenteric artery and its branches usually as far as left colic (splenic) flexure

Small intestine

—— **Efferent fibers**
—— **Afferent fibers**
······· **Parasympathetic fibers**

FIGURE V Vagus nerve (X): Schema

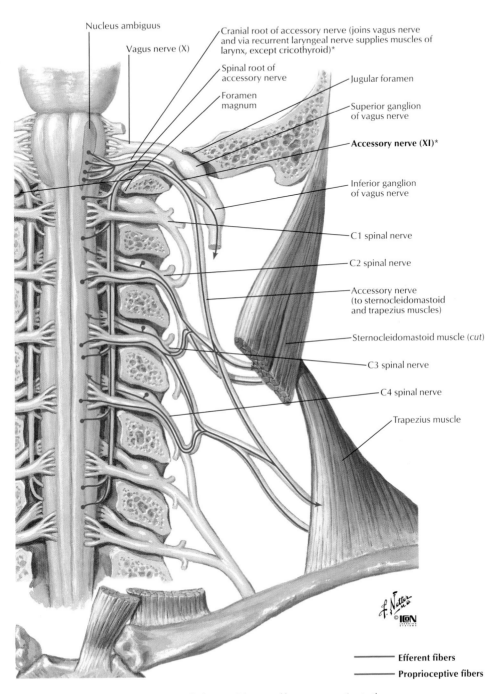

Nucleus ambiguus

Vagus nerve (X)

Cranial root of accessory nerve (joins vagus nerve and via recurrent laryngeal nerve supplies muscles of larynx, except cricothyroid)*

Spinal root of accessory nerve

Foramen magnum

Jugular foramen

Superior ganglion of vagus nerve

Accessory nerve (XI)*

Inferior ganglion of vagus nerve

C1 spinal nerve

C2 spinal nerve

Accessory nerve (to sternocleidomastoid and trapezius muscles)

Sternocleidomastoid muscle (*cut*)

C3 spinal nerve

C4 spinal nerve

Trapezius muscle

——————— **Efferent fibers**

——————— **Proprioceptive fibers**

*Recent evidence suggests that the accessory nerve lacks a cranial root and has no connection to the vagus nerve. Verification of this finding awaits further investigation.

FIGURE VI Accessory nerve (XI): Schema

HYPOGLOSSAL NERVE (XII)

The hypoglossal nerve is mainly a motor nerve; it supplies the muscles of the tongue, except for the palatoglossal muscle, which is innervated by the vagus nerve (X) (Figs. 2.28 to 2.30 and VII). The hypoglossal nerve plays a major role in mastication, sucking, swallowing, and speech.

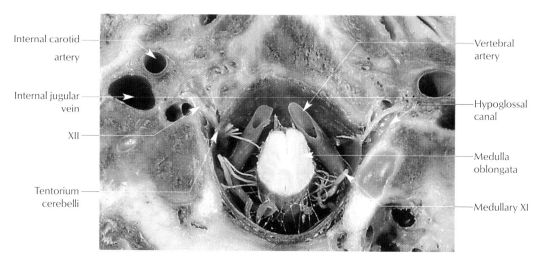

FIGURE 2.28 Axial section overlying the foramen magnum.

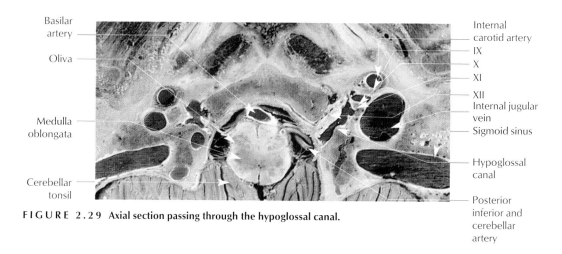

FIGURE 2.29 Axial section passing through the hypoglossal canal.

The ramifications supplying the geniohyoid, thyrohyoid, and infrahyoid muscles are constituted by fibers borrowed from the superficial cervical plexus through a superior anastomosis with the loop of C1, as well as neurofibrilla from the recurrent meningeal ramification and an anastomosis with C2 and C3, which together make up the cervical loop.

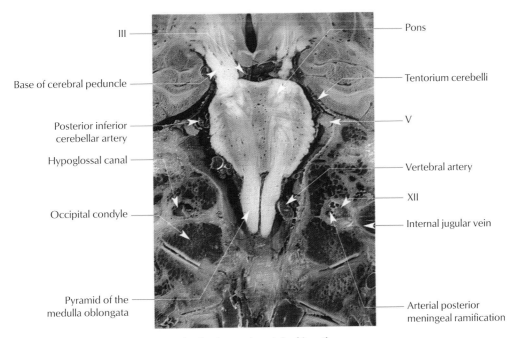

FIGURE 2.30 **Frontal section passing by the craniovertebral junction.**

Pathway

In its canal, the hypoglossal nerve is accompanied by the recurrent meningeal ramification, the meningeal ramification of the ascending pharyngeal artery, and a venous plexus. The hypoglossal nerve travels successively through the lateral pharyngeal space, the carotid trigonum and the suprahyoid region, finally reaching the lateral side of the tongue. In the retrostyloid region, the hypoglossal nerve is deeply situated, behind the internal carotid artery up to the superior cervical ganglion of the sympathetic trunk and the inferior ganglion of the vagus nerve, then sliding forward between the internal carotid artery and the vagus nerve medially and the internal jugular vein laterally. In the carotid trigonum, the hypoglossal nerve curves along the posterior border of the posterior ventral fibers of the digastric muscle and crosses the lateral side of the external carotid artery beneath the origin of the occipital artery. With the internal jugular vein and the thyrolinguopharyngofacial venous trunk, the hypoglossal nerve delimits the classic Farabeuf triangle. In the suprahyoid region, the hypoglossal nerve is attached, with the lingual vein, to the lateral side of the hyoglossal muscle, which separates the hypoglossal nerve and the lingual vein from the lingual artery. The tendon of the stylohyoid muscle and the digastric muscle cross the hypoglossal nerve and the lingual vein laterally. The submandibular fossa is located above.

The hypoglossal nerve slides between the mylohyoid and hyoglossal muscles along the lateral side of the tongue and underneath the submandibular canal before dividing into its terminal branches in the sublingual region, at a distance from the terminal branches of the lingual artery.

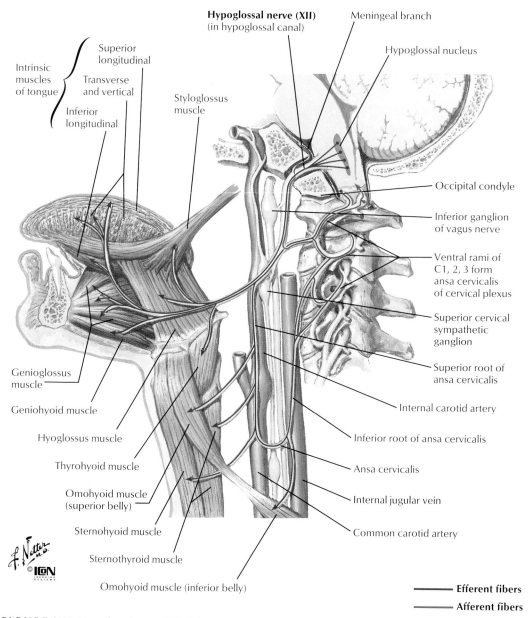

Intrinsic muscles of tongue
- Superior longitudinal
- Transverse and vertical
- Inferior longitudinal

Styloglossus muscle

Hypoglossal nerve (XII)
(in hypoglossal canal)

Meningeal branch

Hypoglossal nucleus

Occipital condyle

Inferior ganglion of vagus nerve

Ventral rami of C1, 2, 3 form ansa cervicalis of cervical plexus

Superior cervical sympathetic ganglion

Superior root of ansa cervicalis

Internal carotid artery

Inferior root of ansa cervicalis

Ansa cervicalis

Internal jugular vein

Common carotid artery

Genioglossus muscle

Geniohyoid muscle

Hyoglossus muscle

Thyrohyoid muscle

Omohyoid muscle (superior belly)

Sternohyoid muscle

Sternothyroid muscle

Omohyoid muscle (inferior belly)

Efferent fibers

Afferent fibers

FIGURE VII Hypoglossal nerve (XII): Schema

Collateral Branches

The collateral branches of the hypoglossal nerve include the **meningeal ramification** borrowed from C1; the **superior root of the cervical loop** formed by fibers from C1, C2, and C3; the **nerve of the thyrohyoid muscle;** and the **nerves of the geniohyoid muscle.**

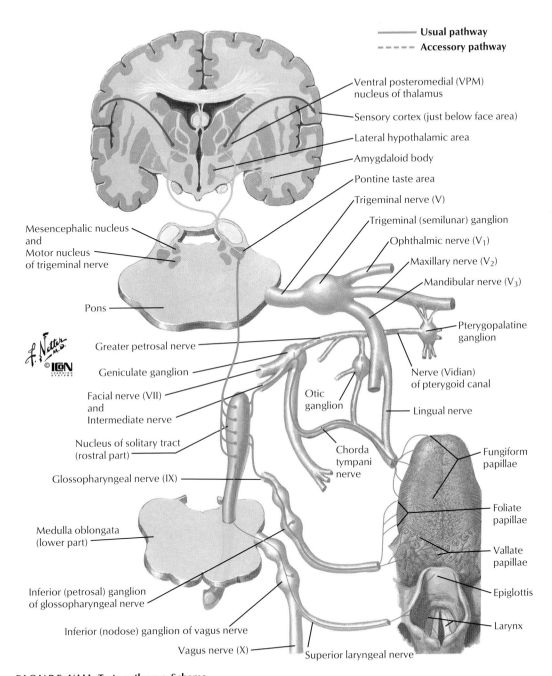

——————— **Usual pathway**
- - - - - - - **Accessory pathway**

Ventral posteromedial (VPM)
nucleus of thalamus

Sensory cortex (just below face area)

Lateral hypothalamic area

Amygdaloid body

Pontine taste area

Trigeminal nerve (V)

Trigeminal (semilunar) ganglion

Ophthalmic nerve (V$_1$)

Maxillary nerve (V$_2$)

Mandibular nerve (V$_3$)

Mesencephalic nucleus
and
Motor nucleus
of trigeminal nerve

Pterygopalatine
ganglion

Pons

Greater petrosal nerve

Nerve (Vidian)
of pterygoid canal

Geniculate ganglion

Facial nerve (VII)
and
Intermediate nerve

Otic
ganglion

Lingual nerve

Nucleus of solitary tract
(rostral part)

Chorda
tympani
nerve

Fungiform
papillae

Glossopharyngeal nerve (IX)

Foliate
papillae

Medulla oblongata
(lower part)

Vallate
papillae

Inferior (petrosal) ganglion
of glossopharyngeal nerve

Epiglottis

Inferior (nodose) ganglion of vagus nerve

Larynx

Vagus nerve (X)

Superior laryngeal nerve

FIGURE VIII Taste pathways: Schema

Terminal Branches

The hypoglossal nerve radiates its terminal branches at the anterior border of the hyoglossal muscle. There, the hypoglossal nerve forms an anastomosis with the lingual nerve.

3

Olfactory Nerve

F. Fuerxer, F. Domengie, and D. Doyon

Olfactory disorders are frequent, disabling, and are often poorly understood or go unrecognized. Olfaction is transmitted by the I nerve, which is part of the rhinencephalon; the nose constitutes the receptor organ of the olfactory clefts. There has been renewed interest in these disorders, which are frequently encountered in certain degenerative diseases (e.g., Alzheimer disease after 40 years, multiple sclerosis).

Because of recent progress in imaging, the olfactory tracts can now be precisely studied. In addition, functional studies of olfaction with MR image (MRI) are in the developmental stage. Frequently, disorders of smell are accompanied by taste disorders (at the worst, ageusia (reduction or absence of the sense of taste), which can be extremely disturbing, especially during the acute phase of viral infections or as an after-effect following severe trauma).

EMBRYOLOGY

Embryologically, the olfactory placodes are located in the nasal fossa (Fig. 3.1). They radiate fibers and cells that combine to form the terminal olfactory and the vomeronasal nerves. These nerves advance cephalad and toward the front through the cribriform plate. When these nerves come into contact with the anterior telencephalic vesicles, they induct the formation of the olfactory bulbs. The bulbs can be individualized after 18 weeks.

ANATOMY
Olfactory Mucosa

The olfactory mucosa is closely applied to the cribriform plate of the ethmoid at the nasal fossa. Yellowish in color, it covers the middle portion of the superior nasal concha and the superior portion of the septum of the nasal fossa for approximately 1 cm at the so-called yellow spot, or olfactory region. Its total surface is approximately 10 cm^2. The olfactory mucosa is composed of a neuroepithelium, a basal lamina, and Bowman tubuloalveolar glands.

The olfactory neurosensorial cells are bipolar protoneurons. They contain a dendrite whose cilium has a membrane that holds the odor receptors. The amyelinated axons of the olfactory neurosensorial cells pass through the basal membrane along with other axons that they have joined, forming the primary olfactory fibers. The primary olfactory fibers penetrate into the cranial cavity through the foramens of the cribriform plate of the ethmoid.

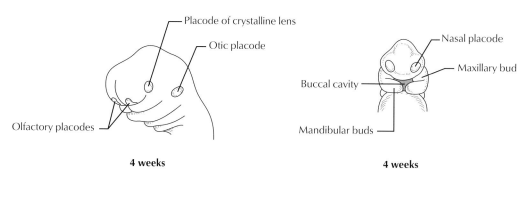

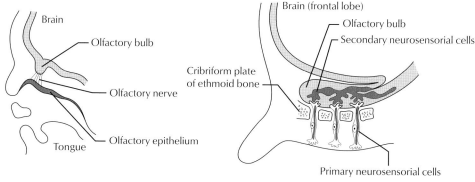

FIGURE 3.1 Embryologic diagrams.
Formation of the olfactory bulb during the first 16 weeks of development.

The Olfactory Bulb

On either side of the crista galli, the cribiform plate is narrow and deeply grooved; it supports the olfactory bulbs (Figs. 3.2 to 3.6). On the orbital surface of the frontal lobe, the olfactory bulbs are beneath the olfactory sulcus, which separates the medial orbital gyrus from the gyrus rectus. The bulb corresponds to the arrival relay of the peripheral neuron and the starting point of the second-order central neuron represented by the mitral cell.

Olfactory Tract and Rhinencephalon

The olfactory tract, prismatic, originates at the posterior pole of the bulb and stretches out onto the basal surface of the frontal lobe in the olfactory sulcus. At its point of insertion on the frontal lobe or the trigonum olfactorium, the olfactory tract divides into three olfactory striae: lateral, medial, and intermediate. The initial portions of the lateral and medial olfactory striae outline, with the bandaletta diagonalis, the anterior perforated substance.

The basal olfactory areas are formed by the gray matter and receive the direct, secondary olfactory projections coming from the central neurons of the olfactory bulb. These areas consist of

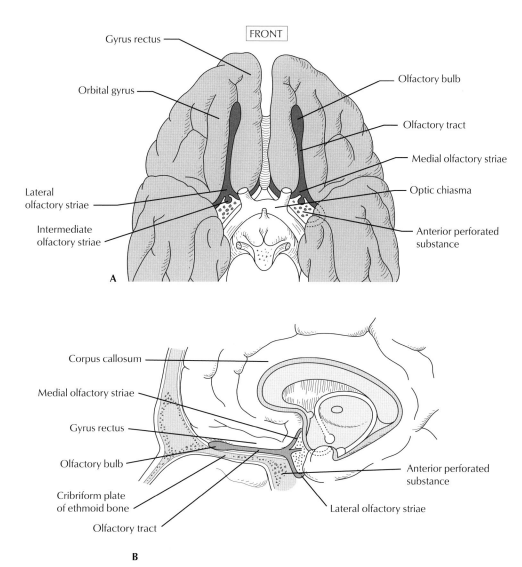

FRONT

Gyrus rectus

Orbital gyrus

Olfactory bulb

Olfactory tract

Medial olfactory striae

Optic chiasma

Lateral olfactory striae

Intermediate olfactory striae

Anterior perforated substance

A

Corpus callosum

Medial olfactory striae

Gyrus rectus

Olfactory bulb

Cribriform plate of ethmoid bone

Olfactory tract

Anterior perforated substance

Lateral olfactory striae

B

FIGURE 3.2 Anatomic views of the olfactory bulbs.
(**A**) Inferior. (**B**) Sagittal.

the following: the anterior olfactory nuclei (located in the caudal portion of the bulb, in the olfactory tract, and in the rostral portion of the olfactory tubercle), the prepiriform cortex, and the cortical nucleus of the amygdaloid body.

The secondary olfactory projections travel exclusively along the lateral olfactory stria. This stria extends laterally, then enters into the middle cerebral fossa by suddenly curving opposite the limen insulae before penetrating into the rostromedial portion of the temporal lobe. The lateral olfactory stria consists of the subcallosal and parateral gyrus area and the limbic system.

The intermediate olfactory stria continues for a short distance along the course of the olfactory tract before plunging into the anterior perforated substance by lifting the olfactory tubercle.

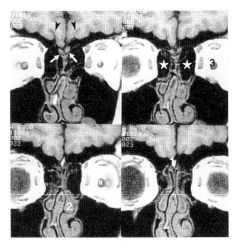

FIGURE 3.3 Normal anatomy.
Series of four 3-mm continuous, T1-weighted
coronal MR image sections from back to front. The
two olfactory bulbs (⇒) are clearly visible and the
two olfactory sulci (➤) are well outlined, analyzed
6 mm behind the Crista Galli during hypersignal (1)
(↗) (★ = ethmoidal cells; 2 = middle concha; 3 =
optic nerve) on anterior sections.

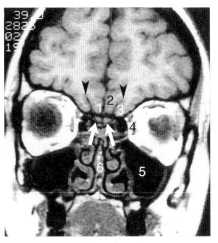

FIGURE 3.4 Normal anatomy.
T1-weighted coronal MR image section. The two
olfactory bulbs (⇒) are visible and the two
olfactory sulci are well outlined (➤) on both sides
of the midline (1) (2 = gyrus rectus; 3 = olfactory
gyrus; 4 = internal orbital lamina; 5 = maxillary
sinus; 6 = nasal septum).

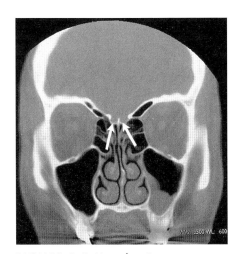

FIGURE 3.5 Normal anatomy.
Frontal computed axial tomography scan sections.
Cribiform plate is narrow and deeply grooved (⇒).

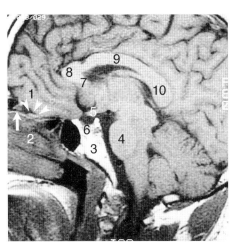

FIGURE 3.6 Normal anatomy.
Three-millimeter paramedian T1-weighted sagittal MR
image sections. One of the two bulbs (➤) is visible
under the frontal lobe (1) during isosignal above the
nasal mucosa (⇒). (2 = middle concha; 3 = clivus;
4 = pons; 5 = optic chiasma; 6 = sella turcica;
7 = rostrum of corpus callosum; 8 = genu of corpus
callosum; 9 = body of corpus callosum;
10 = splenium of corpus callosum).

The tertiary olfactory projections transmit information from the rhinencephalon to the neocortex and the reticulomotor system of the brainstem. Among these projections, the centroposterior orbitofrontal (CPOF) and lateroposterior orbitofrontal (LPOF) cortical regions should be noted. The prepiriform cortex and the medial portion of the amygdaloid body emit afferents by the transthalamic route toward the CPOF (a region that seems to be involved in olfactory discrimination), as well as afferents that travel by the innominate substance (lateral portion) before entering into the LPOF (by the extrathalamic route).

Because of its close relationship to the limbic system, the olfactory tract is involved in the neurovegetative system, emotions, behavior, and related motor responses. In humans, the rhinencephalon is poorly developed compared with certain animals whose olfactory capacities are well known; the polar bear can detect odors at a distance of 6 kilometers and hunting dogs can still distinguish odors a few hours after the stimulus has passed.

ETIOLOGIES OF DISORDERS OF THE SENSE OF SMELL

There are a number of different disorders of the sense of smell: for example, **hyposmia,** or reduced sense of smell, which can result in **anosmia**. **Hyperosmia** is the exaggeration of olfactory perceptions (often extremely unpleasant and termed **cacosmia**). **Parosmia** is a perversion of the sense of smell in which the scent detected does not correspond to the stimulation. Olfactory hallucinations without any stimulating odor are due to a discharge in the orbital surface of the frontal cortex. Finally, olfactory discrimination can be lost and can result in the inability to identify different odors.

These different disorders of the sense of smell can have a number of different etiologies, although the following list is not all inclusive.

Peripheral Lesions

Locoregional

Six can be mentioned:

Nasal polyposis (the most frequent etiology)

Acute viral or bacterial rhinitis

Nonallergic eosinophilic rhinitis (NARES)

Sinusitis

Allergic rhinitis (a rare cause)

Tumor involvement (Fig. 3.7)

Viral

Herpes

Viral hepatitis

Toxic

Most frequent causes:

Tobacco

Benzene

Cement

Ammonia

Cocaine

Medications (nasal sprays, aminoglycerides, tetracyclines, etc.)

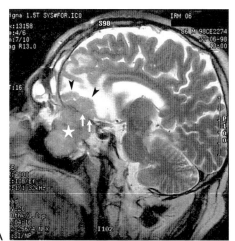
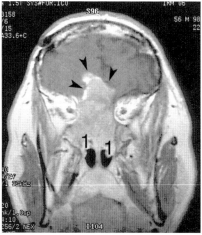

A   B

FIGURE 3.7 Esthesioneuroblastoma.
(A) Sagittal T2-weighted MR image (MRI) section. Voluminous expansive process in the ethmoid–nasal region (★) that has destroyed the cribriform plate (⇒) with endocranial extension and invasion of the frontal lobe (➤). (B) Frontal T1-weighted MRI section with gadolinium injection. Enhancement of the entire tumor extending to the inferior concha (1) and frontal lobes (➤). The orbits are not involved.

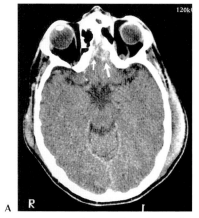
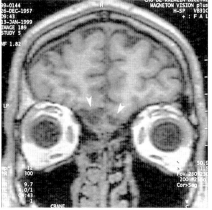

A   B

FIGURE 3.8 Posttraumatic anosmia (and ageusia).
(A) Computed axial tomography scan, axial section, on day 1. Bilateral hyperdense, basifrontal, hemmorhagic contusions are seen (⇒). (B) T1-weighted, 3-mm frontal MR image section. Bilateral residual bands with hyposignal are seen (➤). The bulbs cannot be identified.

Posttraumatic (Fig. 3.8)

The clinician must consider fracture of the anterior floor of the base of the skull with involvement of the cribriform plate. This is characterized as follows:

Usually caused by an occipital shock

In order of frequency: olfactory filaments, nasal and sinus cavities, cerebral centers

Severity depends on the magnitude of the trauma

Immediate or delayed anosmia (progressive meningeal "fibrosis")

Recovery is rare

Postoperative, iatrogenic
> Seen after surgical traction on the frontal lobes

Central Lesions

Central lesions are characterized as follows:

- Frontal or occipital traumas
- Expansive processes (Table 3.1)
- Neurotoxic medications

TABLE 3.1 Expansive Processes

Anterior Floor of the Base of the Skull	*Middle Floor of the Base of the Skull*
Meningioma of the ethmoid	Craniopharyngioma
Meningioma of the small sphenoid wing	Frontal tumor
Meningioma of the olfactory sulcus	Glioma and glioblastoma
Olfactory esthesioneuroblastoma	Oligodendroglioma
	Tumor of the third ventricle
	Hypophyseal tumor
	Tumor of the corpus callosum

Other Causes

Endocrine
> Consider the following:
>> Cushing disease
>> Hypothyroidism
>> Diabetes mellitus

Neurologic
> There are multiple neurologic causes:
>> Alzheimer disease
>> Parkinson disease
>> Korsakoff psychosis
>> Down syndrome
>> Multiple sclerosis
>> Epilepsy
>> Schizophrenia

Congenital (Fig. 3.9)
> Three should be considered:
>> Kallmann de Morsier syndrome
>>> Hypogonadotropic hypogonadism
>>> Small size
>>> Delayed puberty (eunuchism)
>>> Often transmitted by X chromosome

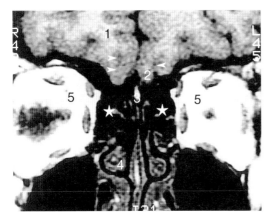

FIGURE 3.9 Kallmann de Morsier syndrome.
T1-weighted coronal MR image section. None of the bulbs is visible. The olfactory sulci (➤) are poorly outlined and are not very deep. (1 = frontal lobe; 2 = gyrus rectus; 3 = Crista Galli; 4 = middle concha; 5 = orbit; ★ = ethmoid cells).

      Isolated congenital anosmia

      Atresia of the choana

Various

    Other possible causes include:

      Alcoholic cirrhosis and hepatic failure

      Renal failure

      Acute acquired immune deficiency syndrome (AIDS)

      Aneurysm of the anterior communicating artery

      Paget disease

Idiopathic

    Usually related to advanced age

CLINICAL WORKUP FOR DISORDERS OF THE SENSE OF SMELL

Patient History

Characterization of the Disorder

The clinician should clarify the following:

    1. The dysosmia: disorder of smell

      A. Quantify it

        1. Hyposmia: reduction in smell

        2. Anosmia: total loss of smell

      B. Qualify it

        1. Parosmia: a false olfactory impression in the presence of a stimulus

        2. Cacosmia: the perception by the patient of a disgusting odor, in the absence of an appropriate stimulus

        3. Phantosmia: olfactory hallucination

        4. Uncinal seizures: disgusting or ghost odors that should prompt the clinician to exclude an internal temporal cerebral lesion

2. Mode of onset
   A. Sudden
   B. Progressive
3. Remarkable patient history
   Look for the following:
   A. Past trauma
   B. Surgical history
      1. Of the nose or sinuses
      2. Of the anterior or middle floor of the base of the skull
      3. Neurosurgery
   C. Medical history (see above).
4. Inquire into spontaneous fluctuations or changes after corticosteroid treatment
   A. These situations should suggest a nasal or sinus disorder
5. Look for nasal clinical signs (30% of adults have altered nasal and sinus function)
   These include:
   A. Nasal obstruction
   B. Rhinorrhea
   C. Sneezing, epistaxis

Physical Examination

Should include the following:

- Endoscopic examination of the nasal cavities
- Complete head, eye, ear, nose, and throat examination
- Neurologic examination
- General examination

Other Diagnostic Procedures

Patients with permanent, persistent disorders of the sense of smell in the absence of an obvious cause should be considered for the following procedures:

- CT scan of the sinuses: this is the first procedure to order and it should be performed without contrast injection if MR image (MRI) is available
- Olfactory testing: not often utilized
- Allergy testing
- MRI: an essential procedure when an expansive process is suspected

Causes That Should Not Be Neglected When a Patient Has a Disorder of the Sense of Smell

- Alzheimer disease after age 40 years
- Multiple sclerosis before age 40 years

■ Past trauma to the anterior floor of the base of the skull (do not forget to systematically include parenchymal windows of the anterior floor with the CT scan)

■ An MRI is indicated when an esthesioneuroblastoma or meningioma is suspected

SUMMARY

Dysosmias or disorders of the sense of smell are divided into the following categories:

1. **Transmission** dysosmias related to the following:

   A. A mechanical nasal obstruction (deviated septum, after-effects following fracture, a benign or malignant tumor, hyperpneumatization of the middle concha)

   B. Inflammation of the nasal mucosa from acute or chronic allergic or vasomotor rhinitis, polyposis, or sinusitis

2. **Perception** dysosmias related to the following:

   A. Lesions in the central olfactory nervous centers (olfactory nerve, olfactory bulb, rhinencephalon, etc.) due to head trauma, neurosurgery, tumor, a toxic cause, or viral infection

   B. Central lesions causing epilepsy and olfactory hallucinations, Parkinson disease, and Alzheimer disease

Optic Nerve (II), Visual Pathways

M. Hadj Rabia, F. Benoudiba, D. Doyon, and H. Offret

OPTIC NERVE

The optic nerve, the second pair of cranial nerves, is formed by approximately 1,200,000 myelinated axons. The optic nerve comprises the first segment of the optic pathways and extends from the posterior pole of the ocular globe to the anterolateral angle of the optic chiasma. The optic nerve does not have the same characteristics as a peripheral nerve because it is an extension of the central nervous system and just like the central nervous system, it is surrounded by a sheath extending from the corticospinal meninges. As a result, the optic nerve can never develop a primary schwannoma or neurofibroma.

Three segments of the optic nerve are individualized: *intraorbital, intracanalar,* and *intracranial* at the level of the optochiasmatic cistern. Beyond the optic chiasma, the fibers are called the optic tracts. They go around the cerebral peduncles before joining the lateral geniculate body, which produces the optic radiations.

Imaging Techniques and Normal Anatomy

Computed Axial Tomography Scanning

Computed axial tomography (CT) scanning is performed with contiguous, 5-mm-thick axial sections extending from the foramen magnum to the orbital floor followed by 3-mm-thick sections up to the orbital roof; the remainder of the brain is explored with 10-mm-thick sections. After injection of iodine contrast material, the thickness of the sections can be modified according to the size of the lesion discovered. High-resolution millimetric sections permit careful analysis of the orifices of the base of the skull and particularly the optic canal in its different planes.

The axial sections must be parallel to the neuro-ocular plane (NOP), which was defined by Cabanis (orbitomeatal plane: 15 to 20°). This allows alignment of the two crystalline lenses, the papillae, and the optic canals from front to back, thus including the entire visual pathway.

Coronal sections are directly performed when there is no contraindication (trauma to the spinal cord) or with multiplane reconstruction using fine, axial sections facilitated by a continuous rotation apparatus.

The optic nerve can be seen within the adipose tissue of the orbit, separated from the muscular cone by the perioptic meninges; CT scanning cannot differentiate between the nerve and the peripheral liquid spaces. The intracanalar segment of the optic nerve is difficult to see because of the partial volume effect induced by the neighboring body structures. The main role of the CT scan is to detect calcifications, notably papillary calcifications, which are characteristic of the drusen. CT scanning is also very useful in traumatology and in exploring bony lesions (Fig. 4.1).

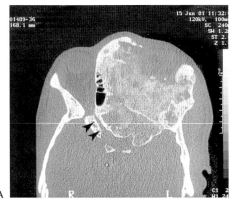

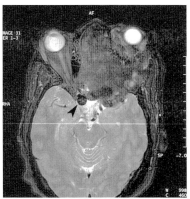

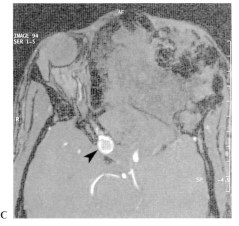

FIGURE 4.1 Blindness in the left eye in a 50-year-old patient.
Recent reduction in vision in the right eye. Fibrous dysplasia (McCune-Albright syndrome) localized in the frontal–ethmoid–sphenoid regions completely narrowing the left optic canal, associated with a right carotid–ophthalmic aneurysm (➤) responsible for the reduced right eye vision (the bony portion of the optic canal is unaffected) (➤➤). **(A)** Computed axial tomography scan, axial section with a bone window passing through the optic canal. **(B)** Turbo spin echo T2 axial MR image section after fat suppressed. **(C)** Angiomagnetic resonance time of flight sequence (native section).

MR Image

When no contraindication is present (any intraocular ferromagnetic foreign body, ferromagnetic cerebral clip, pacemaker) MR image (MRI) is the best technique for exploring the optic nerve. The patient must keep both eyes closed or fixed on a precise point during the time needed for recording the images to avoid artifacts related to movement.

MRI should be performed in an antenna head to enable the totality of the visual pathways to be explored and to look for other associated intracranial lesions. A detailed study of the orbital contents can be obtained with an orbital surface antenna, although its main inconvenience is signal loss in greater depth.

The optic nerve should be studied in a number of different planes because of its tortuous pathway, which allows the ocular globe to move without exerting any traction on its fibers.

Sections in the transhemispheric NOP (THNOP) can be performed (Fig. 4.2). These sections align the optic nerve sagittally, notably its intracanalar segment. These sections also allow visualization of the contralateral calcarine sulcus. Coronal or perpendicular sections in THNOP can also be performed (Fig. 4.2B).

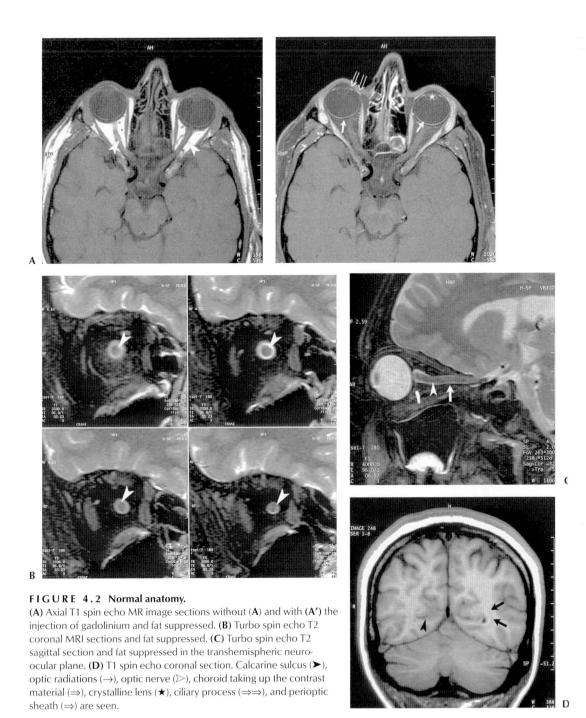

FIGURE 4.2 Normal anatomy.
(**A**) Axial T1 spin echo MR image sections without (**A**) and with (**A′**) the injection of gadolinium and fat suppressed. (**B**) Turbo spin echo T2 coronal MRI sections and fat suppressed. (**C**) Turbo spin echo T2 sagittal section and fat suppressed in the transhemispheric neuro-ocular plane. (**D**) T1 spin echo coronal section. Calcarine sulcus (➤), optic radiations (→), optic nerve (▷), choroid taking up the contrast material (⇒), crystalline lens (★), ciliary process (⇒⇒), and perioptic sheath (⇒) are seen.

T1 spin echo MRI sequences produce good contrast between the optic nerve and the neighboring orbital fat (Fig. 4.2A). T2-weighted MRI sequences and T1-weighted MRI sequences after gadolinium injection using techniques that suppress fat and are very sensitive for detecting abnormal signals and pathologic signal absorption in the optic nerve through an increased signal form of a hypersignal within fatty tissue, which is hyposignal (Fig. 4.3).

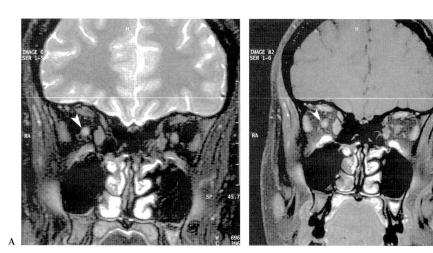

FIGURE 4.3 A 27-year-old woman reported significant reduction in visual acuity with pain on mobilization of the right eye.
Enlarged right optic nerve with hypersignal in T2 taking up gadolinium suggested inflammatory optic neuritis (➤).
(A) Turbo spin echo T2 coronal MR image section with fat suppressed. **(B)** T1 spin echo coronal section after gadolinium injection and fat suppressed.

In MRI, the optic radiations are easily seen (Fig. 4.2D) close to the ventricular bifurcations and the occipital horns, where they appear with a T1 isosignal and a T2 hyposignal from the lateral corpus geniculi to the calcarine sulcus. Because of its transversal orientation, the calcarine sulcus is more clearly visible in the coronal and sagittal planes. The ophthalmic artery around the optic nerve and the ophthalmic vein located above the superior portion of the orbit can also be studied with MRI.

In addition to morphologic sequences, MRI permits the study of the mobility of the optic nerve in the horizontal (NOP) or vertical (THNOP) planes, and thus being able to differentiate a soft tumor (glioma of the optic nerve) from a hard tumor (perioptic meningioma).

Other Techniques

Conventional radiography is sometimes used during the course of certain disorders, particularly during trauma. Orbital Doppler ultrasound is useful essentially for studying the ocular globe and neighboring structures. The posterior portion of the orbit is difficult to study because orbital fat is hyperechogenic.

Lesions

The optic nerve represents a long extension of the brain and its envelopes. For this reason, the majority of lesions that can affect the central nervous system can also be found in the optic nerve (Table 4.1).

TABLE 4.1 Principal Lesions of the Optic Nerve

Optic Neuropathies of Tumor Origin
Gliomas and meningiomas of the optic nerve sheath
Lymphoproliferative processes
Tumors spreading from the ocular globe (retinoblastoma)
Metastases (lung and breast carcinomas in adults, neuroblastomas in children)
Inflammatory or Infectious Optic Neuropathies
Optic neuritis (multiple sclerosis)
Sarcoidosis
Histiocytosis
Inflammatory pseudotumor
Wegener's granulomatosis
Tuberculosis, toxoplasmosis, herpes, human immunodeficiency virus
Vascular and Posttraumatic Lesions

Optic Nerve: Tumors

Glioma of the Optic Nerve

Glioma of the optic nerve is a relatively benign tumor that develops from glial cells (astrocytes, oligodendrocytes). This lesion is mainly encountered in children around age 5 years and corresponds to a low-grade astrocytoma (usually pilocytic, more rarely fibrillar). Optic nerve gliomas in children are often associated with type I neurofibromatosis (Von Recklinghausen disease; NF1). Gliomas in adults are more rare, predominant in women, and are occasionally malignant (glioblastoma).

Gliomas of the optic nerve are slowly progressive tumors that can extend along the optic nerve, causing progressive axial exophthalmia, or towards the perioptic meninges without invading the dura mater. Doppler ultrasound can demonstrate enlargement of the optic nerve.

In gliomas of the optic nerve, CT scanning shows a hypertrophied optic nerve with a variable morphology, either fusiform, truncular, or excentric, that is isodense compared with the uninvolved contralateral optic nerve. The nerve appears homogeneous or contains hemorrhagic areas or intratumoral cystic degenerative zones when it is voluminous; microcalcifications are frequently seen. After injection with an iodine contrast medium, enhancement is variable according to the microscopic picture.

During T1 spin echo MRI, the lesion produces an isosignal or a hyposignal compared with the gray matter (Fig. 4.4). The signal intensity of the lesion is variable during T2-weighted sequences; according to its fibrillary structure or mucoid contents, the signal intensity can vary from weak to intense. With MRI, one can evaluate the degree of tumor spread to the optic canal and detect eventual involvement of the cisternal segment of the optic nerve.

Involvement of the chiasma is seen in NF1, often with dilatation of the perioptic subarachnoid spaces, suggesting dura-submerian dysplasia (Fig. 4.5). Sometimes, abnormal signals are visible along the retrochiasmatic optic pathways in the form of zones with a T2 hypersignal that can correspond to spread from either an optic nerve glioma or a hamartoma. These hamartomas can appear slightly hypersignal during T1 without enhancement after gadolinium injection, without a mass effect on midline structures; these hamartomas remain stable over time and have a tendency to become smaller or even to disappear.

Perioptic Meningoma

Primitive meningiomas specific to the optic nerve are seen mainly in women between ages 30 and 50 years (80% of cases) but can occur in children around age 10 years, in which case they are often

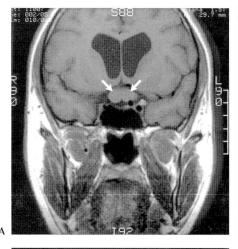

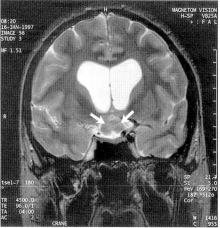

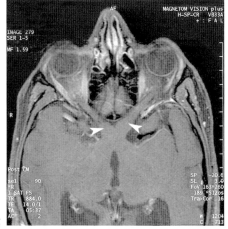

FIGURE 4.4   Reduction in visual acuity in a 48-year-old patient with type 1 neurofibromatosis. Glioma of the chiasma and the optic nerves, which are enlarged (➤ and ⇒). **(A)** T1 spin echo coronal MR image section. **(B)** Turbo spin echo T2 coronal section. **(C)** T1 axial section after gadolinium injection and fat saturation.

associated with neurofibromatosis. Perioptic meningiomas derive from meningothelial cells of the arachnoid and develop either in a circular fashion or excentrically in relation to the axis of the optic nerve.

Perioptic meningiomas are spontaneously hyperdense in CT scanning, with intense enhancement after the injection of iodine. CT scanning can demonstrate intra- or peritumoral psammous calcifications. In T1 spin echo MRI, the lesion appears isosignal or hyposignal compared with the muscular structures surrounding the optic nerve. Like intracranial meningiomas, in T2-weighted sequences the signal is variable as a function of the histologic type. This tumor proliferation intensely absorbs contrast material after injection with gadolinium, closely holding the optic nerve, which remains in hyposignal, thus producing the classic "rail picture"; this aspect can also be observed during CT scanning and during the course of other disorders (optic neuritis, inflammatory pseudotumour, sarcoidosis). MRI can detect perioptic meningiomas and associated intracranial meningiomas (meningiomatosis) at a very early stage.

Spheno-orbital meningiomas and meningiomas of the jugum and/or the tubercle of the sella (Fig. 4.6) can also invade the orbit through the bone, the orbital fissures, and the optic canal. MRI is useful in determining their orbital and temporal extension. Standard radiography and CT scanning can be useful in looking for hyperostosis and associated calcifications.

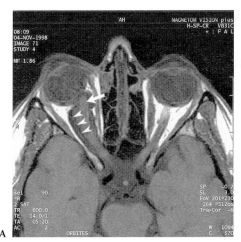
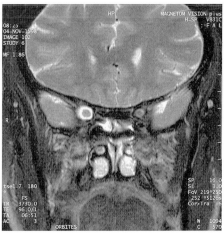

FIGURE 4.5   Significant reduction in visual acuity of right eye in a 43-year-old patient.
Glioma of the right optic nerve with hypertrophy of the nerve (⇒) at its intraconic portion with dilatation of the perioptic sheath (➤). Discrete right exophthalmia. **(A)** T1 axial spin echo MR image section without gadolinium injection. **(B)** Turbo spin echo T2 coronal section.

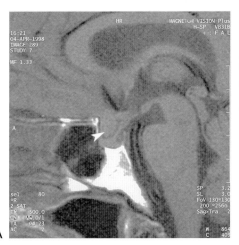
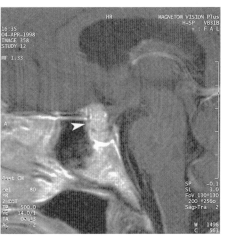

FIGURE 4.6   Visual disturbances in the form of scotomas with superotemporal flattening in the visual field of a 55-year-old patient.
T1 sagittal spin echo MR image section without **(A)** and with **(B)** gadolinium injection. Meningioma of the tubercle of the sella and the diaphragm of the sella (➤).

In addition to perioptic meningiomas and gliomas of the optic nerve, other tumors may be encountered: e.g., hemangiomas, lymphomas, and neurofibromas (III, IV, V, and VI), invade the cavernous sinus, metastases (breast, lung, etc.), which are located mainly in the choroids, ocular tumoral processes extending to the optic nerve (retinoblastoma, melanoma), and aneurysms or infarction (Fig. 4.7).

1. Inflammatory Optic Neuropathies. Demyelinating diseases are the most frequent causes of optic neuritis in adults (multiple sclerosis [MS], de Devic optic neuromyelitis). Targeted MRI (thin sections, THNOP, gadolinium injection) can identify a potentially important diagnostic element, notably in classic retrobulbar optic neuritis, where signal anomalies can be identified: hypersignal in

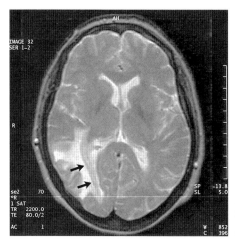

FIGURE 4.7 Left upper quadrant anopsia in a 47-year-old patient.
Vasogenic edema secondary to an optic meningioma involving the optic nerve.

T2 (Fig. 4.3) within a segment of the optic nerve that is increased in size. These anomalies can show increased uptake of contrast material after gadolinium injection when they are in the active phase. MRI can also detect dissemination to the central nervous system. However, imaging is not specific and findings should be correlated with the rest of the clinical and laboratory workup.

A number of other disorders can also involve the optic nerve (sarcoidosis, toxoplasmosis, tuberculosis, dysthyroid neuropathies, inflammatory pseudotumor).

2. Traumatic Lesions. Compression of the optic nerve requires an emergency CT scan to exclude a fracture of the orbital apex or an eventual retro-ocular hematoma or perineural compression. The main value of MRI is to study the intracanalar segment of the optic nerve, the portion that is most vulnerable to trauma because of its adherence to the canal's dura mater. A signal anomaly suggests a centroneuronal contusion at that level (Fig. 4.8).

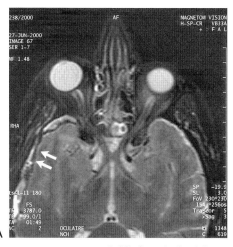
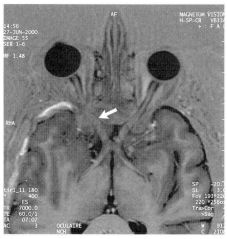

FIGURE 4.8 Posttraumatic blindness in the right eye.
T2 axial turbo spin echo MR image sequences (**A**) and inversion-recuperation sequences (**B**). Contusion of the right optic nerve in its intracanalar segment is seen (⇒). Note obliteration of the perioptic spaces compared with the contralateral side. Subdural hematoma (⇒⇒).

Optic Chiasma

The principal lesions that can compress the optic chiasma are pituitary macroadenomas with suprasellar spread (Fig. 4.9); metastases; craniopharyngiomas; hypothalamochiasmic astrocytomas; meningiomas, notably of the sphenoid jugum, the tubercle of the sella, and/or the diaphragm of the sella (Fig. 4.6); multiple sclerosis, which can also involve the optic nerve, the chiasma, and even the optic bandalettas; and basilar meningitis, notably due to tuberculosis, sarcoidosis (Fig. 4.10), and parasellar aneurysms.

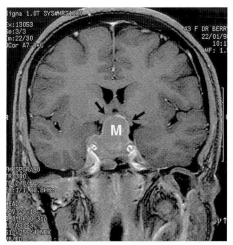
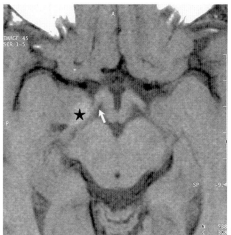

FIGURE 4.9 Acromegaly.
Macroadenoma (M) of the hypophysis with sellar extension eroding the optic chiasma (→). There is a right lateral budding optochiasmic tumor (★) that is impinging on the optic bandaletta (⇒); this tumor is responsible for left homonymous lateral hemianopsia. **(A)** T1 coronal spin echo MR image section after gadolinium injection. **(B)** T1 axial spin echo section.

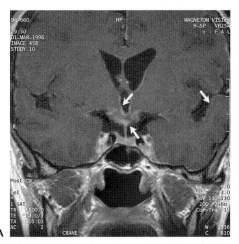
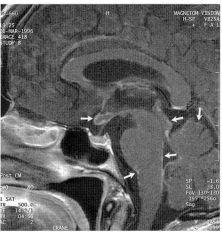

FIGURE 4.10 Granulomatous uveitis with reduction in visual acuity and headaches in a 55-year-old patient.
Coronal section **(A)** and sagittal section **(B)** during T1 spin echo MR image sections after gadolinium injection. Infundibulochiasmic neurosarcoidosis with perichiasmic infiltration and involvement of the leptomeninges of the base of the skull are seen (⇒).

Retrochiasmic Pathways

Cranial hypertension due to tumor or any other etiology (hydrocephalus, diffuse cerebral edema, cerebral pseudotumor, thrombophlebitis) can produce papillary edema, notably in children. This increase in intracranial pressure can be transmitted to the perioptic subarachnoid spaces, which become wider and more tortuous around a normal-sized optic nerve; this aspect is more clearly visible with MRI than with a CT scan. Almost every lesion that involves the optic tracts and the optic radiations between the lateral corpus geniculi and the occipital cortex can produce either homonymous lateral hemianopsia or homonymous lateral quadranopsia (Fig. 4.11).

Ischemic cerebral accidents occur mostly in the occipital cortex (Fig. 4.12). Ischemic cerebral accidents produce a sudden defect in the visual field compared with tumors, which have a progressive onset.

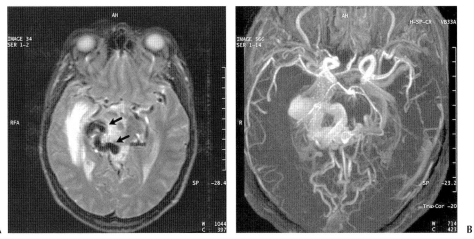

FIGURE 4.11 **Campimetric defect in the form of a left homonymous lateral hemianopsia in a 45-year-old patient.** A right petroclival arteriovenous fistula, which empties into to right sinus through a large right lateromesencephalic vein and which produced a mass effect on the cerebral peduncles, is seen. **(A)** T2 axial spin echo MR image section, second echo. **(B)** Maximum intensity projection magnetic resonance angiography reconstruction after gadolinium injection.

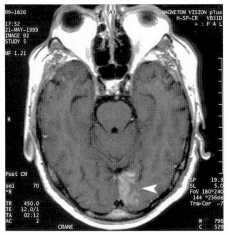

FIGURE 4.12 **Sudden onset of right homonymous hemianopia in a 60-year-old patient.** T1 axial section after contrast. Ischemic accident in the territory of the left posterior cerebral artery (gyriform enhancement of the left internal occipital cortex) (▷).

VISUAL PATHWAYS

The visual pathways begin at the retina and end in the occipital cortex after passing through the optic papilla, the optic nerve, the optic chiasma, the optic tracts and the optic radiations.

The clinical aspects of disorders of the optic pathways are largely based on the study of the **visual field**. The visual field, measured with Goldmann perimetry (perimeter: an instrument used to explore the scope of the visual field) (Fig. 4.13), studies the retina's luminous sensitivity to white light and visualizes the isopters: retinal curves that are isosensitive to white light. The visual field is studied using monocular vision; this field corresponds to the portion of space that is perceived by an eye fixed on a given point.

From this fixed point, the visual field extends 90° in the temporal field, 64° in the nasal field, 63° in the upper field, and 80° in the lower field. Mariotte spot is a zone of scotoma corresponding to the optic papilla, which projects onto the temporal field between 12 and 18° from the fixation point.

Anomalies of the visual field are characteristic of anatomic lesions to the visual pathway (Fig. 4.14). Anomalies of the visual field include scotomas, which are "unseen" zones in the visual field, and amputations in sectors, quadrants, or even hemianopsias or total amputations.

Retina

The retina is composed of two layers: an external layer that is the pigmented epithelium of the retina, and an internal layer, the neuroepithelium, which contains nine internal retinal layers. Light must travel through the eight internal layers before arriving at the photoreceptors: the cones and the rods. The macular cones provide central visual acuity, photopic vision (the sensitivity of the retina to strong light), color vision, and vision in the central visual field. The rods provide the peripheral visual field and scotopic vision (synonymous with night vision: retinal sensitivity to weak light).

After the cones and rods, the *first neurons* are the bipolar cells, followed by the ganglion cells, the *second neurons*. These ganglion cells travel to the optic papilla before traveling to the optic nerve, the chiasma, and the lateral corpus geniculi. Finally, the *third neurons* travel to the occipital cortex near the calcarine sulcus.

Systematization

There is a central macular tractus that comes from the macular cones. The superior and inferior temporal and superior and inferior nasal peripheral fibers end in the entire optic papilla.

Clinical Aspects

All lesions to the macular region and the macular tractus result in central scotoma. All lesions to the retinal fibers or to the optic papilla translate into the amputation of a section of the visual field. All total lesions in the retinal or papillary fibers produce unilateral blindness.

Optic Nerve

Systematization

In the optic nerve, the temporal fibers are lateral and the nasal fibers are medial. The macular tractus is centrally located and is surrounded by peripheral fibers.

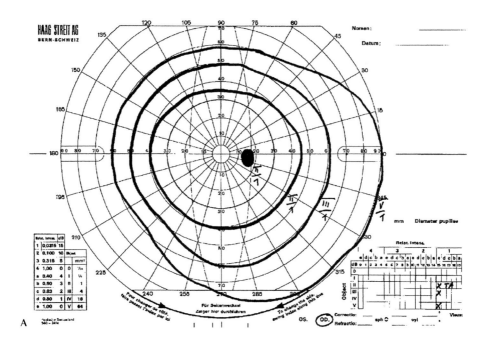

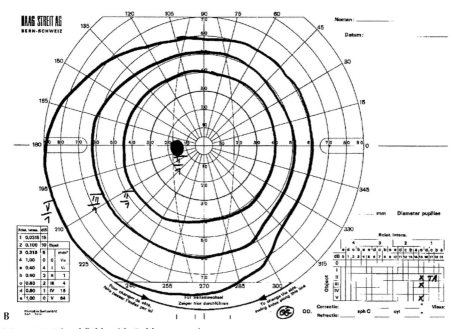

FIGURE 4.13 Visual fields with Goldmann perimetry.
(**A**) Left eye. (**B**) Right eye.

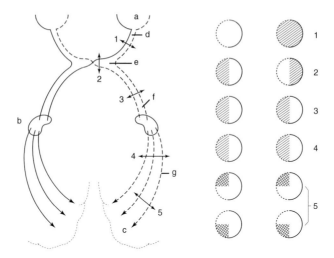

1. Lesion in optic nerve: monocular blindness
2. Lesion in chiasma: bitemporal hemianopsia
3. Lesion in tractus: homonymous lateral hemianopsia
4. Lesion in radiations: homonymous lateral hemianopsia
5. Partial lesions in radiations: homonymous lateral quadranopsia
   - upper if lesion is in lower radiations
   - lower if lesion is in upper radiations

FIGURE 4.14   Diagram of the anatomoclinical relations of a lesion in the optic pathways.
The **(a)** ocular globe, **(b)** lateral corpus geniculium, **(c)** occipital cortex; **(d)** optic nerve, **(e)** chiasma, **(f)** optic tractus, and **(g)** optic radiations are seen.

Clinical Aspects

Section of an optic nerve produces unilateral blindness. A lesion to the macular tractus in the optic nerve elicits central or cecocentral (involving Mariotte spot) scotoma, which is termed central axial neuropathy. Any peripheral disorder of the optic nerve is accompanied by a unilateral sectional amputation of the visual field that is nasal if the lesion is lateral and temporal if the lesion is medial.

Optic Chiasma

Systematization

At the optic chiasma, the temporal fibers are direct and ipsilateral and travel to the optic tract while remaining in a lateral position. The nasal fibers decussate: the fibers from the nasal region, including the fibers from the nasal section of the macula, cross the midline before entering the contralateral optic tract. A portion of these fibers bend near the intracranial extremity of the optic nerve before returning to the chiasma.

Clinical Aspects

A lesion in the *anterior genu* of the chiasma results in one of two possibilities:

- *Blindness* on the same side as the lesion and temporal quadranopsia on the other side.
- *Central scotoma* on the same side as the lesion and quadranopsia on the opposite side; this is termed Traquair scotoma.

All central, longitudinal lesions in the optic chiasma result in classic bitemporal hemianopsia due to an alteration in the decussating fibers of the two nasal fields.

Optic Tract

Systematization

The direct temporal fibers of the optic tract are lateral and the crossed nasal fibers are medial; the central fibers are located in the center of the optic tract.

Clinical Aspects

All lesions to the optic tract result in contralateral, lateral, homonymous hemianopsia with conservation of central visual acuity in both eyes because one half of the macular fibers in both eyes remain untouched by the lesion.

Lateral Geniculate Body

Systematization

The fibers of the optic tract arrive at the lateral geniculate body after twisting; they divide into a number of superimposed layers coming from the ipsilateral and contralateral eye.

Clinical Aspects

Alterations in the visual field are rare and produce lateral homonymous quadranopsia.

Superior Colliculus

The superior colliculus receives a few fibers from the optic tract and the lateral geniculate body. The superior colliculus coordinates eye movements.

Optic Radiations

Systematization

The optic radiations spread from the lateral geniculate body to the occipital cortex. The fibers from the upper part of the retina are above, those from the lower retina are below, and the macular fibers are found in the center. The visual pathways are gathered together at their origin and then divide into two tracts, the superior and the inferior, before coming together once again at the caudal region when they enter the calcarine sulcus.

Clinical Aspects

Lesions in the two anterior or posterior extremities of the optic radiations produce lateral homonymous hemianopsia. A lesion restricted to one superior or inferior portion produces lateral homonymous quadranopsia.

Visual Cortex

Systematization

The visual cortex occupies both borders of the calcarine sulcus on the medial surface of the occipital lobe. The macular fibers occupy an extensive area, spreading to the fundus and along the borders of the calcarine sulcus.

The fibers from the upper retinal quadrants end along the upper border of this sulcus, whereas those fibers from the lower quadrants and along its lower border.

Clinical Aspects

Deficits in the visual cortex consist of either a lateral homonymous hemianopsia or a quadranopsia. In general, the macula is spared.

Nerves III, IV, and VI

M. C. Petit-Lacour, C. Iffenecker, and H. Offret

GENERALITIES

Oculomotor Nerve (III)

Pathway

The oculomotor nerve originates in the cerebral peduncle, near the superior colliculus. The oculomotor nerve emerges from the brainstem in the interpeduncular fossa (Figs. 5.1 and 5.2). The nerve travels along the external wall of the cavernous sinus and then goes through the superior orbital fissure, where it divides into its two terminal branches in the common tendon ring (Zinn ring): an upper branch that travels to the superior rectus muscle and the levator palpebrae superioris and a

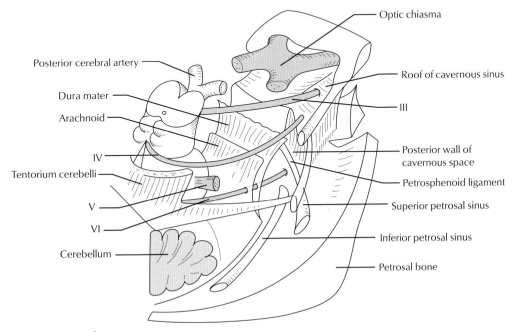

FIGURE 5.1 Oculomotor nerves.
Relationships in the posterior level of the base of the skull.

91

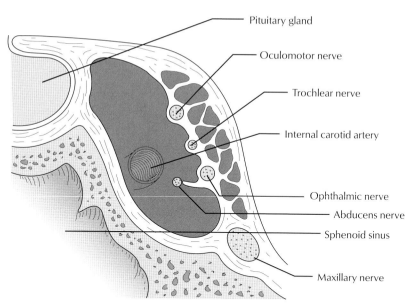

Pituitary gland

Oculomotor nerve

Trochlear nerve

Internal carotid artery

Ophthalmic nerve

Abducens nerve

Sphenoid sinus

Maxillary nerve

FIGURE 5.2 Cavernous space.
Frontal section.

lower branch that travels to the inferior rectus, medial rectus, and inferior oblique muscles. In addition, it contains parasympathetic fibers that travel to the pupil.

Clinical Aspects

Total extrinsic paralysis of the III nerve produces ptosis (and, consequently, the absence of diplopia), external strabismus, and the inability to move the ocular globe upward, downward, or medially. An intrinsic lesion produces mydriasis that does not react to light. This type of mydriasis is usually encountered with lesions to the brainstem and cavernous sinus; otherwise, it is rarely seen.

Trochlear Nerve (IV)

Pathway

The trochlear nerve originates below the preceding nerve opposite the inferior colliculus. The fibers of the trochlear nerve travel backwards, cross the midline, and emerge at the caudal surface of the mesencephalon. The trochlear nerve then travels around the brainstem, passes along the external wall of the cavernous sinus, and then goes through the superior orbital fissure along its thin, external portion before innervating the superior oblique muscle.

Clinical Aspects

Paralysis of the trochlear nerve results in diplopia that is most important downward and in the nasal section. To avoid diplopia, the patient assumes a compensating position: head is inclined and turned toward the unaffected side, with the chin lowered.

Abducens Nerve

Pathway

The abducens nerve (VI) originates in the pontine tegmentum. This nerve emerges at the medial portion of the bulbopontine sulcus and passes over the angle of the petrosal bone. The abducens nerve enters the cavernous plexus through the Dorello canal, a bony canal containing veins and covered by an expansion of the dura mater. The nerve penetrates into the orbit through the superior orbital fissure, in the Zinn ring, and ends directly in the lateral rectus muscle.

Clinical Aspects

Paralysis of the VI nerve results in convergent strabismus in the paralyzed eye. The ocular globe is unable to go beyond the midline and abduct. Sometimes, the patient is able to find a compensating position to avoid diplopia, which is maximal during abduction: the patient turns his or her head toward the paralyzed side, thereby producing eye deviation from the side opposite the diplopia.

Topographic Syndromes

Three types of paralysis have been described:

- Nuclear paralysis: Paralysis of the III nerve, generally associated with vertical paralysis.
- Intra-axial segment: Alternate syndromes.
- Extra-axial segment: Most frequently observed because of the lengthy pathway of the nerves.
  - Interpeduncular syndromes: Double paralysis of the III nerve, double hemiplegia.
  - Syndrome of the cerebellopontine angle: Involvement of the VIII, VII, V1, then VI and eventually III, cerebellar syndrome.
  - Syndromes of the angle of the petrosal bone: Gradenigo-Lannois syndrome (otitic syndrome, neuralgia of the V nerve, paralysis of the VI and VII nerves).
  - Cavernous space syndromes (ophthalmoplegia, disorder of V nerve, slight exophthalmia):
    - Intracavernous syndrome (paralysis of VI nerve before the others)
    - Extracavernous syndrome (paralysis of III nerve, followed by the V and VI)
    - Syndrome of the anterior cavernous sinus (superior orbital fissure syndrome: ophthalmoplegia, deficit of V1 nerve, slight exophthalmia).
  - Orbital apex syndrome: Superior orbital fissure syndrome and optic nerve impairment.

Because of the complex pathways of the oculomotor nerves, the clinical evaluation is important in targeting the most appropriate imaging procedures. Imaging studies of the oculomotor nerves are difficult because of the small size of the nerves and their lengthy pathway, which extends from the brainstem to the orbit. High-resolution studies are necessary and MR image (MRI) remains the most useful procedure. Before performing imaging studies for oculomotor paralysis, general causes, including toxic, deficiency, and metabolic disorders, must be excluded.

IMAGING STUDIES AND NORMAL APPEARANCE OF THE OCULOMOTOR NERVES

MR Image

MRI is the gold-standard procedure for studying the oculomotor nerves. MRI is performed with millimetric slices or, better yet, inframillimetric slices during T2 sequences (constructive interference in steady state, three-dimensional, fast spin echo), or with 2- to 3-mm slices during turbo spin echo T2, and during T1 sequences with and without gadolinium injection and fat suppressed in at least 2 spatial planes. Injection is used according to the suspected underlying disorder.

Computed Axial Tomography Scanning

Computed axial tomography (CT) scanning is useful for exploring bony lesions of the sella turcica, the orbit, and for studying calcifications within tumors. CT scanning is unable to show nerves directly, although their pathways and their exit orifices at the base of the skull can be seen using this modality (Fig. 5.3).

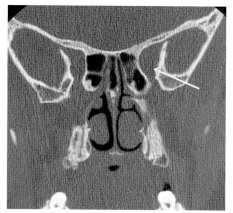
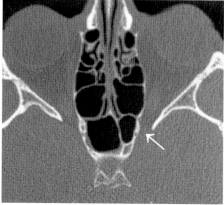

A   B

FIGURE 5.3 Computed axial tomography scan of the base of the skull.
Coronal (**A**) and axial (**B**) sections. Arrow indicates the superior orbital fissure.

The **III,** or the **oculomotor nerve** can be identified in the three spatial planes in the interpeduncular cistern, particularly at the level of the vascular claw, which is constituted by the posterior cerebral artery and the superior cerebellar artery (Fig. 5.4). Coronal sections after gadolinium injection allow examination of the cavernous sinus, with the III nerve located in the superolateral wall of the sinus, lateral to the carotid artery (Fig. 5.5). Farther along, near the superior orbital fissure, the III nerve cannot be seen.

The **IV,** or the **trochlear nerve** is the smallest cranial nerve (0.3 mm). The trochlear nerve is difficult to individualize at its point of emergence beneath the inferior colliculus and in its circumpeduncular pathway, where it merges with the free border of the tentorium cerebelli. Like the III nerve, the cavernous sinus can be studied with coronal sections after contrast injection where the IV follows its course lateral to the internal carotid and beneath the III nerve, with which it merges more often than not. It cannot not be seen near the superior orbital fissure (Fig. 5.5).

The **VI**, or the **abducens nerve** is thin. The abducens nerve can be seen on an axial MRI section at its point of emergence from the bulbopontine sulcus (Fig. 5.6A). In its ascending, prepontine

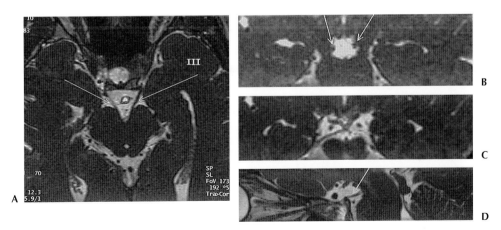

FIGURE 5.4 Normal III nerve.
Constructive interference in steady state sequence with 0.7-mm sections. The III nerve can be seen in the interpeduncular cistern (**A, B, C**) in the claw formed by the posterior cerebral artery (CP) and the superior cerebral artery (ACS) (**C**). Parasagittal reconstructions (**D**) show the III nerve in its subarachnoid and intracavernous portion.

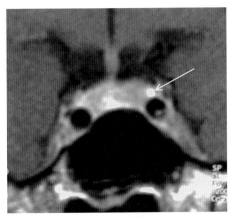

FIGURE 5.5 Anatomy of the cavernous sinus.
T1 coronal sequence after gadolinium injection centered on the cavernous sinus. The III nerve is seen at the superolateral portion of the cavernous sinus (→). The other nerves can be seen from time to time.

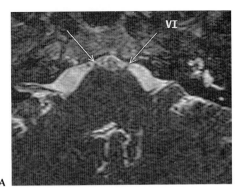

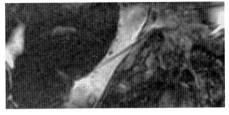

FIGURE 5.6 Subarachnoid pathway of the VI nerve (→).
Axial (**A**) and sagittal (**B**) sections that are 0.7 mm thick. Constructive interference in steady state sequence.

pathway, the abducens nerve can be visualized on sagittal sections (Fig. 5.6B). The abducens nerve passes completely through the dura mater of the dorsum sellae through the Dorello canal, a venous space that is visible in T2 hypersignal (Fig. 5.7). When studying the cavernous sinus with

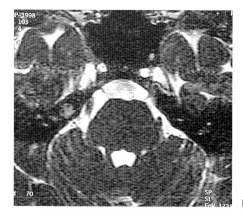

FIGURE 5.7 The Dorello canal (→).

coronal sections after contrast injection, the abducens nerve can be seen traveling along the cavernous sinus, close to the inferior wall of the internal carotid (Fig. 5.5). The abducens nerve cannot be seen near the superior orbital fissure.

CLINICAL ASPECTS

An oculomotor nerve can be damaged at any point from its nuclear origin to its muscular ending (Table 5.1). The patient history, physical examination, and associated disorders of other cranial nerves or of the long pathways can help to localize the lesion. Depending on the results of the clinical

TABLE 5.1 Principal Etiologies of Disorders of Cranial Nerves II, IV, V, and VI in Relation to the Topography of the Lesion

Localization of Lesion	Etiologies
Brainstem segment	Vascular ischemia (SCA thrombosis: infarction of the mesencephalic tegumentum), hemorrhage, malformation (cavernoma); tumors: metastases, glioma of the brainstem, tumor of the IVth ventricle; infectious and inflammatory: abscess, encephalitis, multiple sclerosis (VI), Gayet-Wernicke syndrome.
Cisternal segment	Vascular: aneurysms of the basilar, posterior cerebral, and posterior communicating arteries; tumors: tumor of the cerebellopontine angle, infiltration of the nerve, pinealomas that mainly produce paralysis of the IV nerve, temporal herniation that produces paralysis of the III; infectious: meningitis of the base of the skull (tuberculosis) often producing paralysis of the VI nerve; Gradenigo syndrome (peak of the petrosal bone) associating the V and VI nerves of otitic origin; traumatic: petrosal bone fracture (VI), direct trauma to the tentorium cerebelli (IV).
Cavernous segment	Vascular: aneurysm of the internal carotid, cavernous sinus thrombosis, carotid–cavernous fistula; tumors: pituitary adenoma with invasion of the cavernous sinus, metastasis, mucocele of the sphenoid sinus, meningioma, chordoma, chondrosarcoma.
Superior orbital fissure	Tumors: benign primitive (meningioma +++) or secondary lesion (metastasis), spread from lesions in the base of the skull; traumatic: fracture of the small wing of the sphenoid; infectious and inflammatory: herpes infection, ophthalmic herpes zoster, nonspecific inflammatory granuloma (Tolosa-Hunt syndrome), sarcoidosis.
Orbital segment	Tumors: metastasis, lymphoma, pseudotumor; infectious (cellulites: VI): contiguous sinusitis, mucocele, mucomycosis, and fungal infections.

SCA indicates superior cerebellar artery.

evaluation, a workup for oculomotor paralysis may include a study of the nuclear and fascicular portions of the nerve within the brainstem and of its extra-axial segment (cisternal and intracavernous pathways and route at the level of the superior orbital fissure).

Before performing additional procedures, general causes of oculomotor paralysis should be excluded: e.g., toxic causes (carbon monoxide poisoning, alcohol poisoning, Gayet-Wernicke syndrome), deficiencies (in vitamins B, C, PP), metabolic causes (diabetes mellitus), ophthalmic migraine, Guillain-Barré syndrome. Imaging can contribute little in these clinical contexts.

Also, a number of other disorders (e.g., intracranial hypertension, subarachnoid hemorrhage) can produce oculomotor paralysis of the VI nerve without providing any information for localizing the lesion.

Nuclear and Brainstem Segment

It is impossible to identify the individual nuclei of the cranial nerves because of the lack of contrast with adjacent structures; thus, the anatomic localizations of these nuclei must be learned. The nuclei of the III nerve are located near the cerebral peduncles, in front of and lateral to the mesencephalic aqueduct, at the level of the superior colliculus. The nuclei of the IV nerve are located directly beneath the nuclei of the III nerve, in front of the aqueduct, at the level of the inferior colliculus. The nuclei of the VI nerve are located in the inferior portion of the floor of the IV ventricle.

Various etiologies are responsible:

- **Vascular**: Ischemic, hemorrhagic, malformations (cavernoma, Fig. 5.8). Thrombosis of the superior cerebellar artery (SCA) produces infarction in the mesencephalic tegmentum as well as SCA syndrome (associating IVth nerve paralysis, ipsilateral cerebellar and Horner syndromes, and contralateral hemianesthesia to heat and pain).
- **Tumors**: Metastasis, glioma of the brainstem (Fig. 5.9), tumor in the IVth ventricle.
- **Infectious and inflammatory**: Abscess, encephalitis, multiple sclerosis (Fig. 5.10).

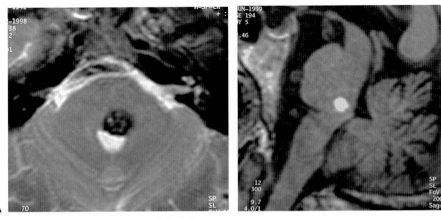

FIGURE 5.8 Cavernoma (paralysis of the left VI nerve).
Axial T2 (**A**) and sagittal T1 (**B**) sequences. Presence of an oval-shaped lesion exhibiting a "salt and pepper" signal during T2 and hypersignal during T1 sequence in front of the floor of the IVth ventricle.

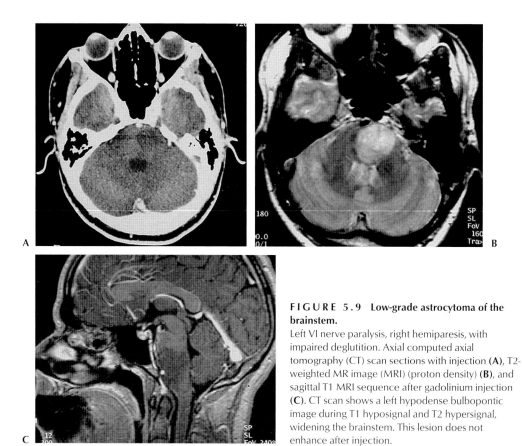

FIGURE 5.9 Low-grade astrocytoma of the brainstem.

Left VI nerve paralysis, right hemiparesis, with impaired deglutition. Axial computed axial tomography (CT) scan sections with injection (**A**), T2-weighted MR image (MRI) (proton density) (**B**), and sagittal T1 MRI sequence after gadolinium injection (**C**). CT scan shows a left hypodense bulbopontic image during T1 hyposignal and T2 hypersignal, widening the brainstem. This lesion does not enhance after injection.

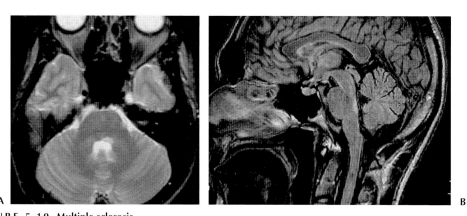

FIGURE 5.10 Multiple sclerosis.

Left VI nerve paralysis. Axial T2 (**A**) and sagittal fluid-attenuated inversion recovery MRI (**B**) sections (→). Area with T2 hypersignal in the anterior portion of the floor of the IV ventricle.

Cisternal Segment

Oculomotor impairment can be isolated after compression by a nearby lesion.

Vascular Etiologies

Most often, aneurysms are responsible for III nerve paralysis due to compression. Aneurysms can be located along the basilar artery, the posterior cerebral artery, or the posterior communicating artery.

Tumor Etiologies

Tumors in the cerebellopontine angle can either compress the III nerve (Fig. 5.11) or infiltrate it (Figs. 5.12 and 6.15B). Particular situations are represented by pinealomas, which produce paralysis of the IV nerve and temporal herniation that produces paralysis of the III nerve.

Infectious Etiologies

Meningitis of the skull base (tuberculosis) is often responsible for paralysis of the VI nerve. Gradenigo syndrome (i.e., lesion located at the apex of the petrosal bone), associated with V and VI nerve impairment, should also be mentioned as a potential infectious cause.

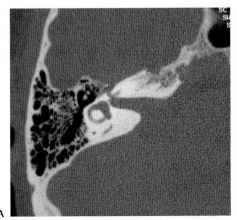

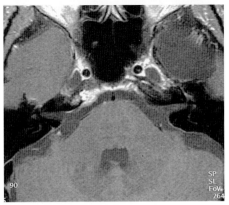

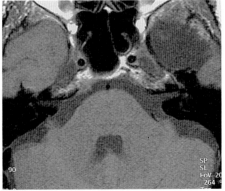

A

B

C

FIGURE 5.11 Meningioma of the petrosal bone. Right VI nerve paralysis. Computed axial tomography (CT) scan section **(A)**. A 3-mm axial T1 MR image (MRI) sequence without **(B)** and with **(C)** gadolinium injection and fat suppressed. The CT scan demonstrates a lytic lesion in the apex of the petrosal bone near the petrobasilar sulcus (in the region of the groove of the VI nerve). MRI during T1 isosignal shows a tissue formation in the parenchyma that enhances after injection and extends to the meninges along a gentle sloping pathway; contrast material is taken up from the meninges to the internal acoustic meatus. The VI nerve (→) is in close contact with this formation. Follow-up 6 months later shows that the lesion has remained stable. The most likely hypothesis is a meningioma is despite the unusual presence of bone lysis.

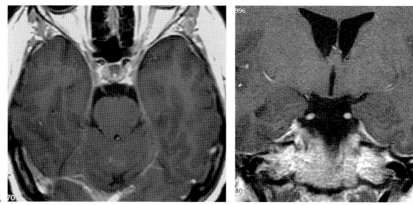

FIGURE 5.12 Metastasis to the leptomeninges with III nerve involvement from a breast cancer.
Spin echo T1 axial **(A)** and coronal **(B)** MR image sections after the injection of contrast material. Contrast material has been taken up by the oculomotor nerves (→) and by the subtemporal meninges.

Traumatic Etiologies

Traumatic etiologies include petrosal bone fracture (VI) and direct contusion of the tentorium cerebelli (IV).

Cavernous Segment

The cavernous sinus syndrome is constituted by lesions of the III, IV, VI, and V nerves. Two main causes: vascular etiologies and pituitary tumors.

Vascular Etiologies

Vascular etiologies of truncal disorders of the intracavernous pathway include:

- Aneurysm of the internal carotid artery (Fig. 5.13)
- Cavernous sinus thrombosis
- Carotid–cavernous fistula (Fig. 5.14)

Tumor Etiologies

Tumor etiologies of truncal disorders of the infracavernous pathway include:

- Pituitary adenomas with invasion of the cavernous sinus (Fig. 5.15)
- Tumor lesions in the cavernous sinus (metastasis, mucocele of the sphenoid sinus, meningioma, chordoma) (Fig. 5.16)

Superior Orbital Fissure Segment

The lesions are revealed by the superior orbital fissure (III, IV, V1, and VI) and orbital apex (III, IV, V1, VI, and optic neuropathy) syndromes. They are located either at the anterior portion of the cavernous sinus or near the superior orbital fissure.

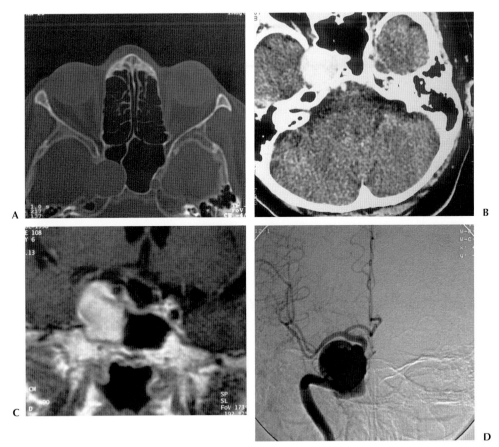

FIGURE 5.13 Right intracavernous carotid aneurysm.
Paralysis of the VI nerve. Axial bone sections (**A**) and axial CT scan following contrast injection (**B**). (**B**) Coronal T1 MRI sequence (**C**), and angiography (**D**). Voluminous right carotid artery aneurysm measuring 3 x 2 cm producing a regular bony deformation of the wall of the sphenoid sinus (**A**). The aneurysm is totally opacified (**B, C**) and, as confirmed by arteriography (**D**), contains no thrombosis.

Tumor Etiologies

- Benign primary (meningioma ++) (Fig. 5.17) or secondary lesion (metastasis)
- Spread from lesions in the base of the skull

Traumatic Etiologies

- Fracture of the small wing of the sphenoid.

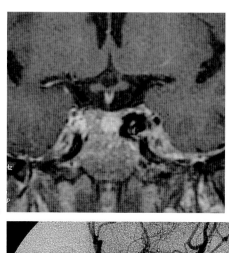

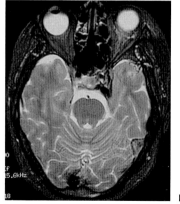

A   B

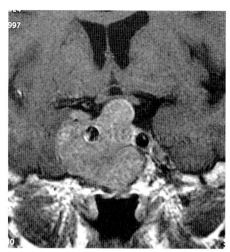

C

FIGURE 5.14 Carotid–cavernous fistula.
Painful exophthalmia with paralysis of the III, IV, and VI nerves. T1 coronal MR image (MRI) section with gadolinium enhancement (**A**) demonstrates dilatation of the left cavernous sinus. T2 axial MRI section (**B**) shows exophthalmia with hyperemia of the orbital fat. Arteriography shows the arteriovenous fistula that opacifies the cavernous sinus.

FIGURE 5.15 Pituitary macroadenoma.
Paralysis of the right III nerve and bitemporal hemianopsia. Coronal T1 MR image sequence with gadolinium injection. The macroadenoma has spread toward the infrasellar region with lysis of the base of the skull (→). Above, there is spreading with filling of the optochiasmic cisterns and compression of the chiasma (➤). Laterally, there is invasion of the cavernous sinus, explaining the oculomotor paralysis and tumor spread surrounding the carotid artery.

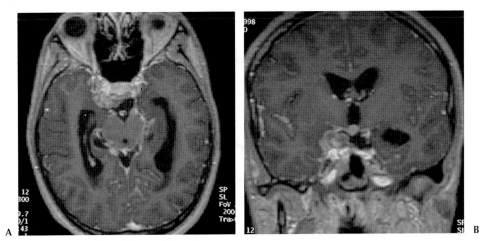

FIGURE 5.16 Metastasis to the cavernous sinus.
Diplopia and right III nerve paralysis in a patient with a high-grade oligodendroglioma that was resected. Axial (A) and coronal (B) T1 MR image sequences with and without gadolinium injection. Tissue process centered in the right cavernous sinus explains the oculomotor paralysis with spread to the sellar region and infiltration of the pituitary stalk and the floor of the III ventricle. Diffuse contrast uptake by the leptomeninges related to a leptomeningeal relapse.

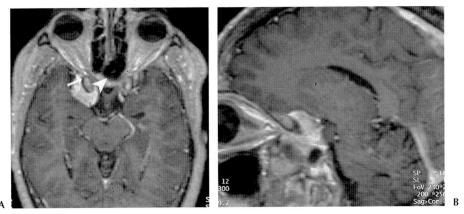

FIGURE 5.17 Meningioma in the small wing of the sphenoid.
Axial and sagittal T1 MR image sequences after injection (A, B). Tissue process in the right small wing of the sphenoid, partially obstructing the superior orbital fissure (→), resulting in a mass effect on the optic nerve (➤).

Infectious and Inflammatory Etiologies

- Herpes infection, ophthalmic herpes zoster
- Nonspecific inflammatory granuloma of one or both cavernous sinuses (anterior portion) (Tolosa-Hunt syndrome) (Fig. 5.18)

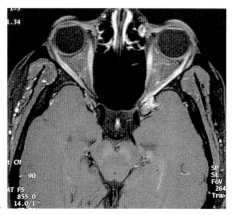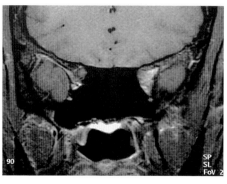

FIGURE 5.18 Tolosa-Hunt syndrome.
Paralysis of the left III, IV, and VI nerves with hemicrania. Axial (**A**) and coronal (**B**) spin echo T1 MR image sequences with fat suppressed. Contrast uptake in the left paracavernous meningeal region and at the superior orbital fissure (→). These anomalies rapidly regressed after corticosteroid therapy.

Orbital Segment

Truncal disorders at the level of the orbit include both tumor and infectious etiologies.

Tumor Etiologies

- Metastasis, lymphoma
- Inflammatory pseudotumour

Infectious Etiologies

- Cellulitis: early, preferential impairment of the VI nerve
- Contiguous sinusitis, mucocele
- Mycomycosis and fungal infections

CHAPTER 6

Trigeminal (V) Nerve: Workup for Trigeminal Neuralgia

K. Marsot-Dupuch

The **trigeminal (V) nerve** is the thickest cranial nerve. It is the nerve of the first branchial arch and carries sensory and motor fibers to the face (Fig. 6.1). Trigeminal nerve impairment requires that the nerve be studied from the brainstem to its most distal branches. Clinical examination is not very useful in localizing the lesion. Impairment of the V1, V2, or V3 can be caused by a nuclear lesion. Associated impairment of other cranial nerves can help localize the lesion (Table 6.1).

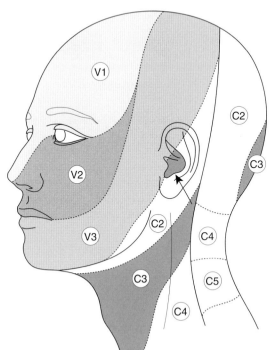

FIGURE 6.1 Facial sensory innervation.
Territories of the branches of the trigeminal nerve: the angle of the jaw and occipital region are innervated by the branches of the superficial cervical plexus; the concha (Ramsay-Hunt area) is innervated by sensory fibers of the VII nerve (→).

TABLE 6.1 Neurologic Syndromes Associated With Impairment of the V Cranial Nerve

Localization	Nerves Involved	Name	Most Frequent Cause
Cerebellopontine angle	V, VII, VIII, sometimes IX	CPA syndrome	Schwannoma, meningioma, tumor of the petrous bone
Apex of petrosal	V, VI	Gradenigo syndrome	Petrositis and tumor of the apex of the petrous bone
Lateral wall of the cavernous sinus	III, IV, V1, ± V2, VI	If inflammatory syndrome: Tolosa-Hunt	Aneurysm/thrombosis of cavernous sinus
Superior orbital Fissure	III, IV, V1, VI	Foix	Invasive tumor of the sphenoid sinus, aneurysm, inflammatory granuloma, invasive sellar tumor

The patient physical examination can be helpful: thus, hypoesthesia of the extremity of the chin is always pathologic and suggests a lesion along the pathway of the V3 nerve. The study of the V cranial nerve can be divided into four segments: the brainstem, the prepontic cistern, the trigeminal cavum and cavernous sinus, and the peripheral branches. Each of these regions has its own specific etiologies that must be ruled out. In addition, the V nerve has numerous anastomoses with the VII and IX cranial nerves that can produce simultaneous impairment of these nerves as well.

IMAGING PROTOCOL

MRI is the first procedure to perform and should study the following:

- The **entire brain**: T2-weighted FLAIR sequence or axial T2-weighted sequence using 4- to 5-mm sections; sagittal T1-weighted sequence using thin sections to analyze the cranial cervical junction.
- The **cisternal pathway of the V nerve and the nuclear region**: High-definition (512) axial SE T2-weighted sequence using 2- to 3-mm sections (Fig. 6.2) from the anterior clinoid processes (upper portion of the trigeminal cave) to the inferior border of the mandible; T1-weighted sequences before and after contrast, with 2- to 4-mm contiguous sections or separated by 1- or 2-mm axial and coronal sections, using a coronal incidence from the brainstem to the ocular globe (Fig. 6.3); CISS gradient echo sequences, thanks to the high signal intensity of the CSF, and submillimetric sections are essential for studying cisternal neurovascular conflicts (Fig. 6.2B and C).
- The **sagittal sequences** unfold the nerve along its long axis and allow the study of its relationship to the petrous apex.
- **Fat-suppressed T1-weighted sequences** identify enhancement of a nerve segment surrounded by fat and demonstrate perineural infiltration.

CT scanning (spiral CT with multiplanar reconstruction) aids in analyzing the walls of the skull base foramina and the bony canals through which the branches of the V cranial nerve pass (Fig. 6.4); it is useful in trauma cases or when the physician is not sure whether a cortical bone segment is intact. CT can demonstrate spontaneous dehiscence in the infraorbital canal along the maxillary sinus or can reveal calcifications if they are present.

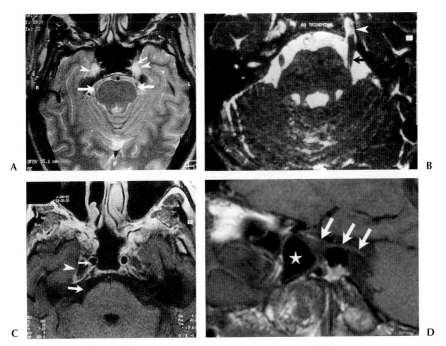

FIGURE 6.2 Cisternal pathway of the V nerve.
Magnetic resonance image, cisternal pathway (arrow) of the V nerve and trigeminal cave (➤). T2-weighted turbo spin echo **(A)** and gradient echo **(B)** showing the branches of the triangular plexus of the trigeminal ganglion (→). T1 sequence after gadolinium injection **(C)** showing the relationships of the trigeminal cave (➤) with the vertical portion of C5 of the carotid siphon (→) medially; sagittal T1-weighted sequence through the prepontic cistern **(D)**, showing the trigeminal nerve and cave (↙↙↙) and the pneumatized pterygoid process (★).

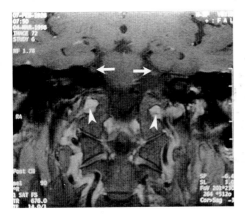

FIGURE 6.3 Cisternal pathway of the V cranial nerve.
Coronal 3-mm T1 spin echo MRI section passing through the prepontic cistern. Pathway of the V cranial nerve in the CPA (→) passing above the plane of the acoustic-facial bundle. The XII cranial nerve is clearly seen in the hypoglossal canal (➤). Pathway of the V cranial nerve (→) crossing the apex of the petrous bone above the acoustic-facial bundle.

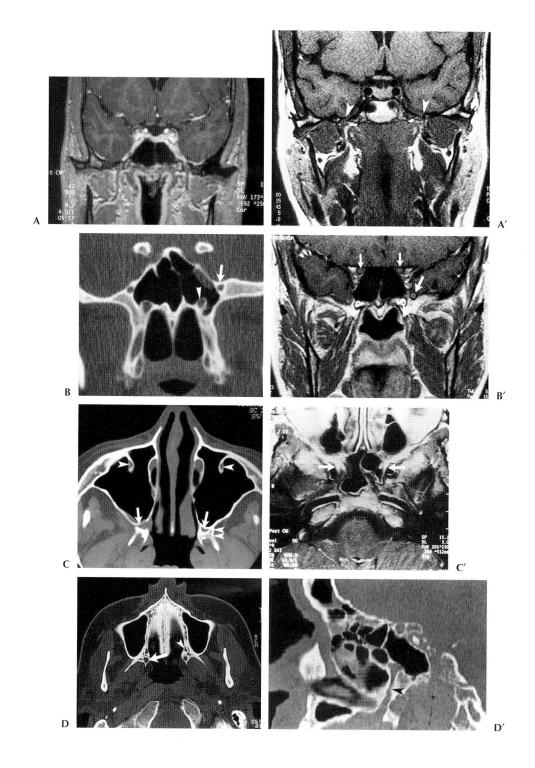

FIGURE 6.4 Comparison of CT scan and MR imaging for the analysis of the peripheral branches.
(A, A′) Foramen ovale (➤), posterior section. The branches of the V3 nerve pass in the infratemporal fossa medial to the lateral pterygoid muscle **(A′)**. Note remodeling of the left sphenoid bone with narrowing of the foramen by a meningioma **(A)**. **(B, B′)** Foramen rotundum (→) and pterygoid canal (➤) **(B)**. Middle section passing through the sphenoid. These canals filled with fat present a high signal intensity in T1-weighted images. This is abolished during sequences with fat suppressed. Note that the optic canal is visible medial to the anterior clinoid processes (arrow) **(B′)**. **(C, C′)** The pterygoid fissure located between the pterygoid process (➤➤) and the palatine (→). Axial CT scan section **(C)**. The infraorbital canal (➤) is visible in the maxillary sinus, opening up in the jugal fossa. MRI section **(C′)** through the pteryopalatine fossa and the foramen rotundum (→). **(D, D′)** Axial CT scan showing the greater (arrow) and lesser (➤) palatine foramens. **(D)** Sagittal CT scan reconstruction through the greater palatine canal (➤), opening into the pterygopalatine fossa. The nerves supply innervation to the palate and provide communication between the oral cavity and the palate and the pterygopalatine fossa.

← *(figure appears on facing page)*

BRAINSTEM

The V cranial nerve presents three sensory nuclei in the brainstem in addition to a pontic motor nucleus innervating the masticatory muscles controlled by the contralateral corticospinal tract. The sensory bulbospinal nucleus, which descends down to C2, carries heat and pain sensation; the mesencephalic nucleus, proprioception; and the pontic nucleus, epicritic sensibility. The nuclei are located in the floor of the IVth ventricle, in its anterolateral portion (Fig. 6.5).

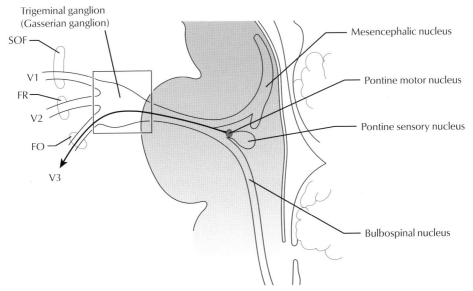

FIGURE 6.5 Distribution of the nuclei of the V cranial nerve in the brainstem and its different branches.
Division of the trigeminal nerve (adapted from Hardin CW, Harnsberger HR: The radiographic evaluation of trigeminal neuropathy. *Semin Ultrasound CT MR* 1987; 8: 214–239). Dividing branches of the trigeminal are as follows: the V1, toward the superior orbital fissure (SOF); the V2, toward the foramen rotundum (FR) and the pterygopalatine fossa; and the V3, toward the oval foramen (OF).

The principal causes of nuclear impairment of the V nerve are listed in Table 6.2:

- **Multiple sclerosis**: Forty percent of patients with multiple sclerosis have a trigeminal neuropathy and Vth nerve impairment is one of the first signs of the disease in 10% of the cases (Fig. 6.6).

TABLE 6.2 Brainstem Lesions That Can Produce Trigeminal Neuropathies

1. Multiple sclerosis	5. Vascular disorders
2. Glioma/metastasis	Arteriovenous malformations
3. Rhombencephalitis	Cavernoma
4. Syringohydromyelia	Infarction
	Dissection

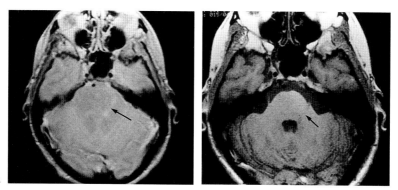

A   **B**

FIGURE 6.6 Nuclear lesions inaugurating multiple sclerosis.
Abnormal visibility of the internuclear pathway of the V nerve in T2 hypersignal **(A)** and T1 hyposignal **(B)** (→).

- **Ischemic vascular accidents** occur most often secondary to small artery disease (high blood pressure), and more rarely to dissection of the basilar artery; ischemic vascular accidents should be considered when complete Vth nerve neuropathy appears suddenly. Vascular disorders can be the cause of residual trigeminal neuropathy long after an acute accident. Gradient echo sequences are useful for demonstrating scars following a hemorrhagic cerebrovascular accident (cerebral vascular malformations that have bled).

- **Rhombencephalitis** (Fig. 6.7) caused by a retrograde brainstem lesion from herpes simplex infection originating in the trigeminal ganglion or secondary to pathogenic infection from microorganisms that have a preferential tropism (listeriosis).

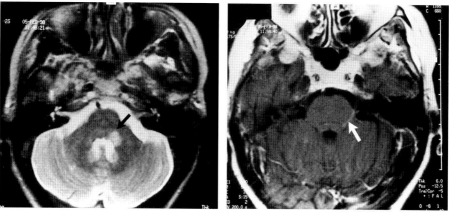

A   **B**

FIGURE 6.7 Viral rhombencephalitis appearing after a herpes labialis infection with diplopia, tinnitus, and sensory impairment of the left side of the face.
(A) T2-weighted sequence through the internal acoustic meatus. Note the presence of a hyperintense, left paraventricular formation (→). **(B)** T1-weighted sequence after gadolinium injection. Note enhancement of the internuclear pathway of the V nerve (→).

DISORDERS OF THE CISTERN OR THE PREGANGLIONIC SEGMENT

The cisternal segment of the V nerve follows an anteroposterior pathway that can be studied using T2-weighted sequences in the axial plane and T1 sequences with and without contrast injection (axial, coronal, and sagittal sections) (Figs. 6.2 and 6.3). The most frequently encountered disorders are due to vascular loops, tumors, and inflammation (Table 6.3). Because the motor and sensory portions of the V nerve are separate, motor and sensory impairment can be dissociated.

TABLE 6.3 Etiologies of Cisternal Disorders of the V Nerve

1. Vascular	4. Tumor
Neurovascular loop	Local
Aneurysm	Neurinoma, neurofibroma (NF2)
Arteriovenous malformation	Meningioma
Dissection of the intrapetrous internal carotid artery	Epidermoid cyst
2. Infectious	Lipoma
Herpes, borreliosis	Regional
3. Inflammatory (meningeal disorders)	Spread from a cavernous sinus tumor
Sarcoidosis, leptomeningeal carcinosis	Tumors of the base of the skull and the apex of the petrosal bone
	Perineural diffusion
	Carcinosis

Vascular Causes

A vascular loop is associated with more than 70% of cases of facial neuralgia or essential facial neuralgia. The vascular compression is due to an arterial crossing: a branch of the superior cerebellar artery (80%), of the anteroinferior cerebellar artery (20%), a venous crossing involving the superior petrosal vein located along the superoexternal border of the nerve (Fig. 6.8), or a mixed crossing, both arterial and venous. The conflict is located at the junction between the central and peripheral myelin, a few millimeters after the exit of the V nerve from the pons, occasionally in the trigeminal cavum. Imaging procedures for the preoperative workup of vascular loops should aim to rule out a cerebral cause (see multiple sclerosis, above), or an aneurysm impinging on the nerve (Fig. 6.9). The study of vascular loops should be performed with MRA and T2-weighted sequence using thin sections (CISS or turbo SE) including oblique and sagittal axial reformations (Figs. 6.8 and 6.10). Low-flow blood vessels can be studied with three-dimensional time-of-flight angiography sequences after gadolinium injection. T1 sequences with gadolinium injection are useful in studying veins that have

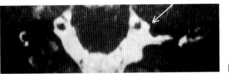

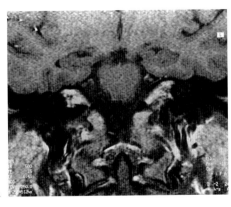

FIGURE 6.8 Vascular loop. Frontal plane.
(A) T1 sequence after gadolinium injection. **(B)** T2 sequence: the nerve is crossed by the superior petrosal vein (→).

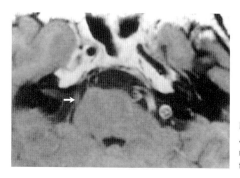

FIGURE 6.9
Aneurysm of the vertebral artery that compresses the trigeminal nerve at its exit point (compare to the normal contralateral trigeminal nerve) (→).

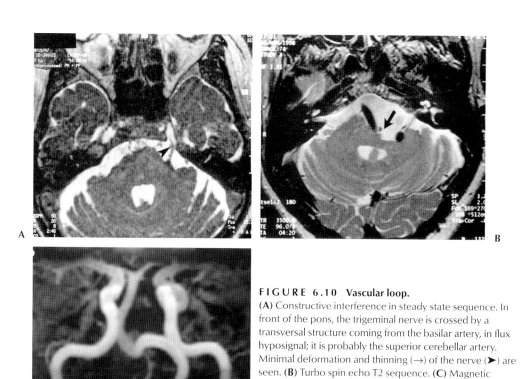

A

B

C

FIGURE 6.10 Vascular loop.
(**A**) Constructive interference in steady state sequence. In front of the pons, the trigeminal nerve is crossed by a transversal structure coming from the basilar artery, in flux hyposignal; it is probably the superior cerebellar artery. Minimal deformation and thinning (→) of the nerve (➤) are seen. (**B**) Turbo spin echo T2 sequence. (**C**) Magnetic resonance angiography. Dolichomegabasilar artery compressing the nuclei of the V and VII nerves on the left.

crossed the nerve (Fig. 6.8). Despite recent technical advances, if a vascular loop is not seen, that does not mean it is not there; the diagnosis is based mostly on clinical criteria.

Tumor Causes

Schwannomas

Schwannomas of the V nerve are rare tumors that develop in the cistern (30%), in the trigeminal ganglion (50%), or simultaneously overlap the posterior cerebral fossa and the cavernous sinus. Schwannomas follow the axis of the nerve and have smooth outlines, a homogenous signal, and

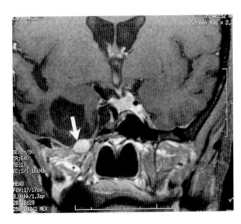

FIGURE 6.11 Relapse of a neurinoma of the V cranial nerve. Coronal section through the anterior portion of the foramen ovale; T1-weighted sequence after injection. Scar resulting from the temporal surgical approach consisting of intraparenchymatous hypointensity. Nodular enhancement of the anterior portion of the foramen ovale (→) is seen.

are relatively hyperintense during T2 MRI (Fig. 6.11). Patients with schwannomas can remain asymptomatic.

Meningiomas

Meningiomas frequently encountered in women in the fifth decade of life. The signal of a meningioma is isointense with respect to normal parenchyma during T1 and T2 sequences; meningiomas demonstrate intense enhancement after gadolinium injection (Fig. 6.12). "Comet tail" enhancement of the dura is frequently associated (65% of the cases); however, even though comet tail enhancement strongly suggests a diagnosis of meningioma, this is not characteristic of the tumor. Two forms of meningioma are described: circumscribed and meningiomas "en plaque." Their severity is due to bone involvement and perineural infiltration along the nerve sheaths. This infiltration allows the tumor to spread toward the fatty spaces at the base of the skull.

Epidermoid Cysts

Epidermoid cysts are rare tumors (fewer than 1% of all intracranial tumors), accounting for 9% of all tumors of the PCA. Epidermoid cysts are characterized by a signal close to that of CSF, except during gradient echo sequences, diffusion sequences, or fluid-attenuated inversion recovery sequences, where they demonstrate a characteristic tissue signal. They have very suggestive lobular outlines (Fig. 6.13). Epidermoid cysts must be differentiated from arachnoid cysts, which have a signal identical to CSF in all sequences, particularly in gradient echo FLAIR and diffusion sequences.

Lipomas

Lipomas are embryonic residues of the primitive meninges; their signal is characteristic: isointense to fat during T1 and T2 sequences. They surround the nerve and the blood vessels, thus rendering their surgical excision difficult.

Metastatic Lesions

Metastatic lesions are due to perineural tumor spread, hematogenous diffusion, leptomeningeal spread or lymphomas (Fig. 6.14). The diagnosis is based on a number of elements: the presence of a known cancer (head, eye, ear, nose, and throat), perineural expanding mass with irregular "fringed" borders, persistent images of nervous system involvement during follow-up examinations, impairment in other cranial nerves, or the presence of enhancement of the dura (Fig. 6.14).

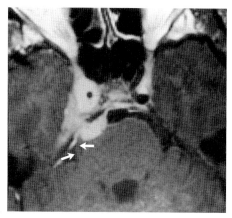

A

FIGURE 6.12 Perineural spread of a meningioma involving the middle and the CPA.
Meningioma overlapping the cistern and the cavernous sinus, pushing the cisternal V nerve laterally (→) and wrapping around the intracavernous carotid, the diameter of which is reduced (A). Meningioma with perineural spread toward the base of the skull, the great sphenoid wing, and the infratemporal fossa. Meningioma of the temporal fossa invading the cavernous sinus, the foramen ovale (B) (➤), and the foramen rotundum (C) (→).

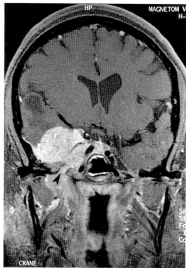

B

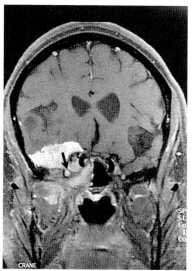

C

Histologic examination of the CSF is positive in 60 to 80% of the cases (at least three microscopic studies should be performed before concluding the examination is negative).

Other Disorders

Inflammatory or viral disorders, whether isolated or in addition to a granulomatous disease, can produce transitory enhancement of the nerve, which keeps its regular outline and habitual diameter (see Fig. 6.15). Most often, the results from examination of the CSF confirm the diagnosis.

DISORDERS OF THE TRIGEMINAL GANGLION AND THE CAVERNOUS SINUS

The V nerve arrives in the trigeminal cave (Meckels cave) after having traveled through the trigeminal incisure of the apex of the petrosal by passing through an orifice, the trigeminal porus. The trigeminal ganglion is surrounded by the leptomeninges, which isolate a cavity of CSF, forming the

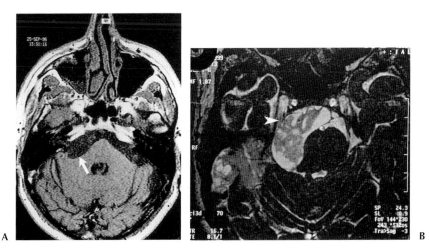

FIGURE 6.13 Epidermoid cysts.
(A) T1-weighted axial section: hypointense lesion (→) in the CPA, slightly lobular, with no contrast uptake and a signal similar to that of cerebrospinal fluid. **(B)** Another patient. An epidermoid cyst recurrance. T2 gradient echo sequence showing a large mass in the prepontic cistern with a heterogeneous signal extending along a cisternal V cranial nerve up to the trigeminal cave (➤).

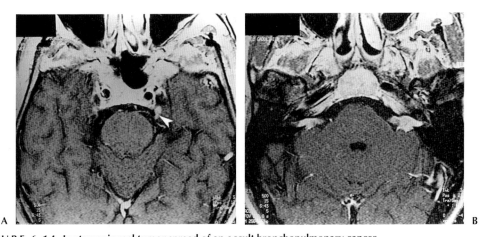

FIGURE 6.14 Leptomeningeal tumor spread of an occult bronchopulmonary cancer.
Facial paralysis and dysesthesia. Axial T1-weighted sequence after gadolinium injection. Abnormal enhancement (➤) of the left trigeminal nerve is seen in the cistern **(A)**. Bilateral expanding masses with irregular contours are seen in the IAMs (internal auditory meatus) **(B)**.

trigeminal cave. Sometimes there are Meckel's megacaves or, on the contrary, hypoplastic caves in cases of congenital paralysis.

The principal branches of the V nerve begin in the trigeminal caves:

- The **V3,** or **mandibular nerve,** which is vertical, exits immediately from the base of the skull through the foramen ovale, where the motor and sensory branches of the V nerve pass. As soon as the V3 nerve enters the infratemporal fossa, it divides into a meningeal branch, a sensory ramification for the tympanic membrane and the external acoustic meatus, and into two motor ramifications: masticators, masseteric branches for lateral

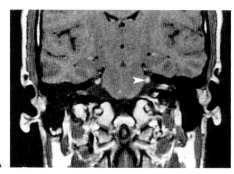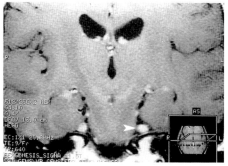

FIGURE 6.15 Lyme disease.
(A) Patient presented with left peripheral facial paralysis. T1-weighted sequence with coronal section. Enhancement of the left acoustic-facial packet, the two V nerves (➤), and the two IV nerves (✓) (asymptomatic). **(B)** Another patient. Lymphomatous tumor of the cistern. Bilateral involvement of the V (➤) and the IV nerves (✓) are seen.

and medial pterygoid, and temporal muscles as well as branches to the tensor veli palatini and the tensor of the tympanic membrane (originating in the branch of the medial pterygoid), and to the myohyoid muscle and the anterior belly of the digastric muscle. The V3 nerve anastomoses with branches of the IX nerve coming from the otic ganglion and with the branches of the VII nerve by the chorda tympani, which innervates the concha of the ear (Ramsay-Hunt area), the external acoustic meatus, and the tympanic membrane. The V3 nerve ends in the inferior alveolar nerve, which follows a mandibular route and takes part in the sensory innervation of the lower portion of the face, except for the angle of the jaw, which is innervated by the branches of the superficial cervical plexus (C2). The foramen ovale constitutes the surgical approach for neurolysis or thermocoagulation of the trigeminal nerve. Otalgia results when its auriculotemporal branch is involved.

- The **V2 nerve,** or maxillary nerve, which is vertical, is the lowest element in the cavernous sinus. The V2 nerve travels under the ophthalmic and the VI nerves before entering the round foramen; it then travels to the pterygopalatine fossa. The V2 nerve ends in the infraorbital nerve, which emerges at the upper portion of the cheek at the base of the canine teeth (Fig. 6.16). The pterygopalatine fossa is a key anatomic area uniting a number of territories: the maxillary sinus by the infraorbital canal; the nasal fossa by the pterygopalatine ganglion; the apex of the petrosal bone by the greater petrosal nerve (pterygoid canal); the palate by the greater and lesser palatine nerves; and the nasopharynx by the pharyngeal ramification of the V2 nerve.

- The **V1 nerve,** or ophthalmic nerve, the most extensive nerve, takes an oblique cephalad route through the superior orbital fissure in the orbit. It divides into three branches: the nasociliary (corneal reflex), the lacrimal, and the frontal, which travels up to the levator palpebrae superioris muscle.

The principal lesions of the V nerve in the trigeminal cavum and its branches in the cavernous sinus are shown in Table 6.4:

- **Intrinsic lesions:** Intrinsic lesions develop from the meninges, the nerve sheath, or from epithelial inclusion.

- **Extrinsic lesions:** Extrinsic lesions develop from continuous tumor spread or by perineural spread (cancer of the cavum: diffusion along the V3 and V2 nerves) (Fig. 6.17).

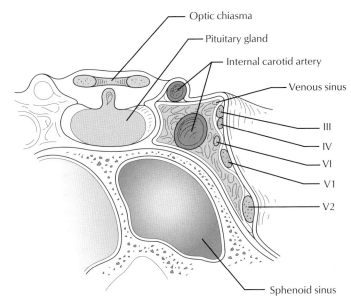

FIGURE 6.16 **Pathway of the branches of the V nerve in the cavernous sinus.**
Section of the sphenoid sinus through the middle portion of the cavernous sinus. The V2 nerve is seen at the lower portion of the cavernous sinus, passing through a split in the dura mater. The V1 passes above the VI nerve. The VI nerve is located under the III and IV nerves, laterally to the VI. The VI nerve is the only one of the oculomotor nerves that travels directly into the cavernous sinus.

TABLE 6.4 Disorders of the V Nerve in the Trigeminal Cavum and the Cavernous Sinus

1. Lesions proper to the trigeminal cavum 　Schwannomas 　Meningiomas 　Epidermoid or arachnoid cysts 2. Lesions invading the trigeminal cavum 　Perineural spread 　Hematogenous spread 　Leptomeningeal spread	3. Intrinsic lesions: 　Chordomas 　Chondrosarcomas 　Bone metastasis 4. Lesions proper to the cavernous sinus 　Spread from a pituitary adenoma 　Aneurysm 　Septic thrombosis of the cavernous sinus

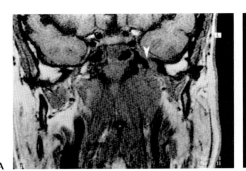
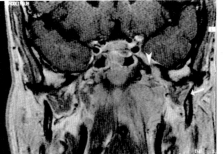

FIGURE 6.17   **Perineural diffusion through the foramen ovale from a nasopharyngeal cancer to the cavernous sinus.**
A 3-mm-thick, T1-weighted MR image scan, coronal section **(A)** and after gadolinium injection **(B)**. Hypointense filling of the foramen ovale (➤) spreading to the cavernous sinus, infiltrating the origin of the mandibular nerve, enhancing after gadolinium injection. An expanding mass is seen in the prevertebral muscles; enhancement of the left lateral pterygoid muscle (→) is also seen, probably secondary to acute denervation.

- **Intracavernous** and **cisternal lesions:** Intracavernous and cisternal lesions develop near the sinus by spread from a pituitary tumor (Fig. 6.18), from an internal carotid aneurysm, or from a pseudoaneurysm that indicates a mass syndrome with characteristic flow void images. When sepsis is present, there is a risk of parietal rupture and vascular exclusion should be suspected when treatment with antibiotics does not lead to improvement. The same is true in cases of epistaxis or when the diameter of an aneurysm increases between two successive examinations, considering the risk involved (Fig. 6.19).

- **Ischemic lesions:** Ischemic lesions develop from damage to the perineural vascularization at the apparent origin of the branches of the V nerve (V1 in the superior orbital fissure, V2 in the round foramen, V3 in the oval foramen). Ischemic lesions mostly involve the inferolateral branch coming from the C4 portion of the intracavernous carotid artery.

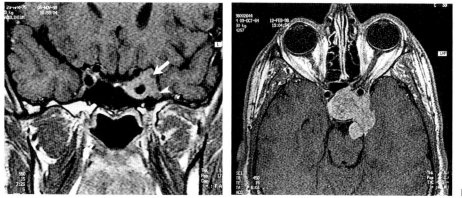

FIGURE 6.18 Pituitary adenoma that has spread to the cavernous sinus, with dysesthesia of the cheek.
T1-weighted MR image sequence after gadolinium injection. **(A)** Coronal section. Deformation of the floor of the sella turcica with tumor invasion into the cavernous sinus around the internal carotid artery, which maintains a normal blood flow. The nervous pathways are surrounded and are seen as round, hyposignal areas. The V2 nerve is located in the lower portion (➤), whereas the III nerve is located in the upper portion (→). **(B)** Another patient, axial section. Spread from a pituitary adenoma into the trigeminal cavum and the mesencephalic cistern.

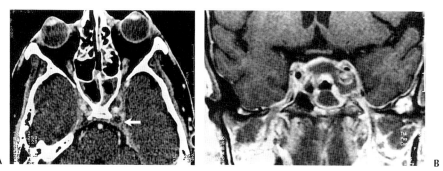

FIGURE 6.19 Septic thrombosis of the cavernous sinus complicated by a pseudoaneurysm of the carotid with rupture.
(A) T1-weighted MRI sequence after gadolinium injection, on admission to the hospital. On the left, widening of the cavernous sinus, which is hypodense (→), is seen. Sphenoid sinusitis. **(B)** Fifteen days later. Enhanced coronal MRI section through the foramen ovale showing the abnormal size of the left internal carotid artery. Persistent anomalies are seen in the pituitary region and the cavernous sinus.

PERIPHERAL DISORDERS

Secondary neurogenic tumors are the most frequently seen, with primary lesions (schwannomas, neurofibromas) being more rare (Fig. 6.20). Involvement of the V nerve is most often secondary to perineural spread or to a metastasis. Perineural spread should be included in workups for upper respiratory malignancies because these malignancies can be associated with tumor diffusion toward the base of the skull and may require a modification in the therapeutic regimen, with surgery or radiotherapy used only for palliative treatment. This involvement can occur simultaneously with the responsible tumor or can precede or follow the responsible tumor by a number of years. Perineural spread can be retrograde or antegrade, diffusing to the nerve branches far from the tumor or even present intervals of tumor-free areas (Fig. 6.21). Tumors that are associated with perineural diffusion along the V nerve include cutaneous tumors (forehead, eyelid for the V1 nerve; cheek, palate, cavum for the V2 nerve [Fig. 6.22]); tumors of the lip, gums, nasopharynx, and intratemporal fossa for the V3 nerve (Fig. 6.17); salivary tumors (cystic adenoid carcinoma [cylindroma] of the palate) that develop along the palatine branches of the V2 nerve; and tumors of the parotid and the submaxillary gland for the V3 nerve.

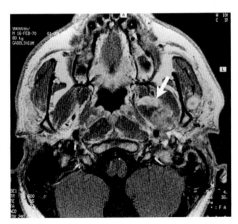

FIGURE 6.20   Neurofibromatosis type II discovered in a patient presenting with swelling of the external acoustic meatus. Multiple masses of varying sizes are seen with nodular enhancement extending to the infratemporal fossa (interpterygoid region) (➤) and the masseter.

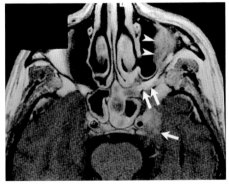

FIGURE 6.21   Perineural spread along V2 with an uninvolved interval. This axial sequence passing through the pterygopalatine fossa following gadolinium injection shows abnormal enhancement in an enlarged infraorbital canal (➤➤), cavernous sinus (→), and cisternal portion of V while the pterygopalatine fossa (→→) has a normal signal.

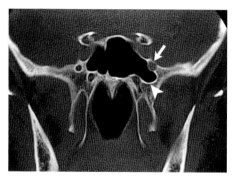

FIGURE 6.22 **Perineural diffusion to the branches of the V2 nerve secondary to a surgically treated melanoma of the cheek.** Coronal computed axial tomography scan. On the left widening of the round foramen (→) and the pterygoid canal (➤) is seen, whose density is greater compared with the contralateral side. Minimal cortical bone loss. (Figure reproduced with the permission of Dr. Gayet de la Croix).

Distal disorders of dental origin are important to recognize. They occur preferentially in apical granulomas or cysts involving the terminal branches of V2 or V3 cranial nerves. Pulpitis constitutes a true emergency with intense pain resistant to analgesics.

Nerve anastomoses can facilitate the involvement of distant nerves and can clinically mimic a polyneuritis (Table 6.5). Anastomoses of the parasympathetic branches of the V1, VII, and IX nerves innervate the parotid gland, the lacrimal glands, the nasal cavity, the pharynx, and the distal two thirds of the tongue and can explain simultaneous involvement of the V and VII nerves. The anastomoses are located near the pterygopalatine ganglion, where the fibers supplied by the greater petrosal nerve (VII) enter the pterygoid canal.

TABLE 6.5 **Anastomoses of the V Nerve**

Nerves	Branches	Anastomosis	Location
Lingual	V3	Sensory VII Chorda tympani	Infratemporal fossa
Auriculotemporal	V3	Secretory VII	Parotid
V2	V2	Greater petrosal nerve (VII), IX	Pterygopalatine ganglion
Otic ganglion	V3	IX, lesser petrosal nerve	Infratemporal fossa

The signs of perineural infiltration include the following:

- Loss of perineural fat (T1) (Fig. 6.23)
- Perineural enhancement (T1 sequence following the injection of contrast material, fat suppressed) (Fig. 6.17)
- Widening and erosion of the bony canal of the nerve (Fig. 6.22)

Signs of motor denervation may be present in cases of injury to the V3. They are separated into the three following phases:

- **Acute phase** with thickened muscles in T2 hypersignal (Fig. 6.24)
- **Subacute phase** with thickened muscles enhancing following contrast material (Fig. 6.25)
- **Chronic phase** with atrophy and fatty infiltration of the muscles (T1 hypersignal)

Traumatic injury to a branch of the V nerve is most often due to imprisonment of the nerve in the fracture site (Fig. 6.26) or to compression by a hematoma. These injuries require CT scan studies of the entire pathway of the V nerve. More rarely, trigeminal neuropathy can be seen after

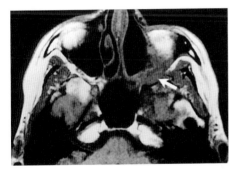

FIGURE 6.23 Perineural diffusion of a cystic adenoid adenocarcinoma treated with surgery and radiotherapy 3 years prior.
Signal anomaly is seen in the pterygopalatine fossa and in the foramen rotundum (→), whose fatty signal has disappeared (compare to the normal contralateral side).

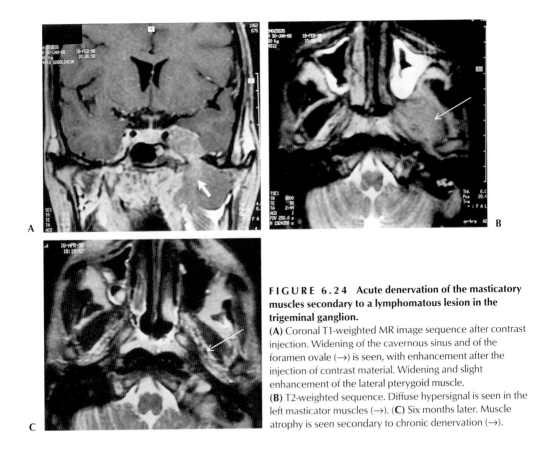

FIGURE 6.24 Acute denervation of the masticatory muscles secondary to a lymphomatous lesion in the trigeminal ganglion.
(A) Coronal T1-weighted MR image sequence after contrast injection. Widening of the cavernous sinus and of the foramen ovale (→) is seen, with enhancement after the injection of contrast material. Widening and slight enhancement of the lateral pterygoid muscle.
(B) T2-weighted sequence. Diffuse hypersignal is seen in the left masticator muscles (→). **(C)** Six months later. Muscle atrophy is seen secondary to chronic denervation (→).

barotrauma to the maxillary sinus with any visible fracture. Trigeminal neuropathy is secondary to ischemia of the nerve predisposed to congenital bone dehiscence. It is most often transitory.

Finally, the physician should remember that the area of the cervical C2 root is projected onto the angle of the jaw. Therefore, cervical C2 root injury may mimic a mandibular nerve lesion. A spinal imaging study should be performed if the cervical root lesion is under discussion.

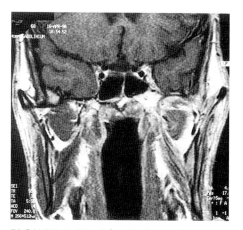

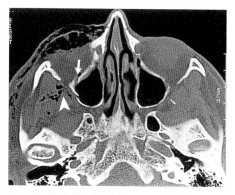

FIGURE 6.26 Facial trauma with injury to the V2 nerve.
Subcutaneous emphysema of the cheek and infratemporal fossa (➤). Collection of air within the infraorbital canal (→).

FIGURE 6.25 Subacute denervation.
Atrophy of the left medial and lateral pterygoid muscles enhancing after gadolinium injection.

CONCLUSION

Imaging studies for a neuropathy of the V nerve should explore the entire pathway of the trigeminal nerve, from its origin to its ending (Fig. 6.27). When the clinical picture includes disabling, progressively worsening pain that is resistant to treatment with analgesics, a tumor origin should be suspected. Negative studies for tumor do not exclude an infraclinical tumor that may have gone undetected for technical reasons, including thickness of study sections, centering of the procedure, or spatial resolution. When sufficient clinical doubt persists, the procedures should be repeated.

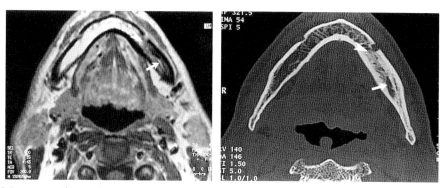

FIGURE 6.27 Injury to the inferior alveolar nerve.
Hypoesthesia of the tuft of the chin leading to the discovery of a chronic aseptic osteomyelitis of the mandible.
(A) T1-weighted MR image sequence after gadolinium injection demonstrating an abnormal signal of the horizontal branch of the mandible (➤) and abnormal enhancement of the inferior alveolar canal (→). **(B)** CT scan, bone window. Sclerosis of the mandible (→) is seen with widening of the inferior alveolar canal (→). Patient was cured with antibiotic therapy.

7

Facial Nerve (VII)

M. Elmaleh-Berges and T. Van Den Abbelle

Most of this chapter explains the differential diagnosis of the peripheral facial paralyses (PFP). The facial nerve is the cranial nerve that has the longest intraosseous pathway: the facial canal. It is important to understand the complex anatomy of the facial nerve to localize the causal lesion and thus determine the etiology of a facial paralysis.

The majority of PFPs are idiopathic. Bell palsy is the most important cause of PFP. However, Bell palsy is a diagnosis of exclusion, after first eliminating all other etiologies by clinical examination and functional testing. Imaging is only indicated when the initial presentation suggests another cause, when the clinical course is atypical, or when surgical decompression is considered.

TOPOGRAPHIC AND FUNCTIONAL ANATOMY

The facial nerve (VII pair) is formed by two roots. One root has a motor function, whereas the other is sensitive, sensory, and secretory, forming the intermediate nerve (Wrisberg nerve) or the VII bis. Pertaining to the motor function of the facial nerve, the cell body of the axons are located in the brainstem; in the case of the sensitive, sensory, and secretory functions of this nerve, the bipolar cells are located in an extra-axial relay ganglion and have two axons, one traveling from the nerve's peripheral origin to the ganglion and the other traveling from the ganglion to the brainstem.

Motor Root of the VII Nerve

The motor nucleus of the VII nerve is located in the lower portion of the pons, lateral to the motor nucleus of the VI nerve. The VII nerve receives fibers from the motor cortex of the two hemispheres. The motor cortex receives information from the paracentral cortex and projects it using the corticospinal tract and consequently, via the posterior arm of the internal capsule:

- Toward the contralateral pontic nucleus solely for the fibers that innervate the lower portion of the face; and
- Toward the ipsilateral and contralateral pontic nuclei for fibers that innervate the upper part of the face.

Consequently, a central or supranuclear facial paralysis spares the upper facial territory.

The fibers from the motor nucleus travel toward the floor of the IVth ventricle, go around the nucleus of the VI nerve, and emerge in the bulbopontine sulcus between the VIII nerve laterally and the VI nerve. In the cerebellopontine trigone, the nerve advances obliquely and laterally and slightly upwards and towards the front, in the direction of the internal acoustic meatus (IAM), the motor fibers covering the sensory fibers. At the far end of the IAM, the VII nerve penetrates the facial canal, which has a complex pathway, in bayonet, in the petrosal pyramid (Fig. 7.1). The first portion of the facial canal, the labyrinthine, 3- to 4-mm long, overhangs the inner ear; after first taking a 75° angle toward the back (genu) and the formation of the ganglion geniculi. The second portion of the facial canal is the tympanic portion, which is 12- to 13-mm long and travels along the medial portion of the tympanic cavity above the window of the vestibule, beneath the lateral semicircular canal. The third portion of the facial canal is the mastoid portion, which is 15- to 20-mm long and is formed after the canal takes a second, 90- to 125° angle (elbow) downward and descends between the antrum and the mastoid cells. The nerve emerges at the base of the skull by the stylomastoid foramen and travels anteriorly, penetrating into the parotid fossa, where it divides into two terminal branches.

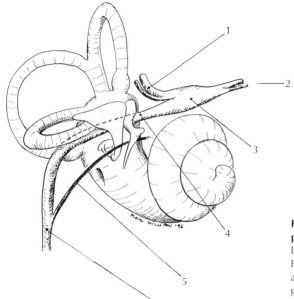

FIGURE 7.1 The facial canal in the petrosal pyramid.
Drawing by Dr. Marc Williams (A. de Rothschild Foundation). 1 = Labyrinthic segment. 2 = Greater and lesser superficial petrosal nerves. 3 = Ganglion geniculi. 4 = Tympanic segment. 5 = Chorda tympani. 6 = Mastoid segment.

In its pathway within the petrosal bone, the VII nerve radiates a motor branch for the stapes; on exiting the skull, it radiates two motor branches: one for the stylohyoid muscle and the other for the posterior belly of the digastric muscle.

In the parotid gland, the nerve divides into its two terminal branches: **superior, temporofacial** and **inferior, cervicofacial**.

VII Bis or Intermediate Nerve

The **VII bis**, or **intermediate nerve** contains sensitive and sensory fibers as well as vegetative or secretory fibers destined for the spinal, solitary, lacrimal, and superior salivary nuclei located in the pons. These fibers, which transmit the sensitivity of the external acoustic meatus, the concha of the auricle (Ramsay-Hunt area) and the retroauricular skin, as well as taste sensation from the distal two thirds of the tongue, use the lingual nerve and the chorda tympani to travel to the ganglion geniculi. Fibers exiting the ganglion geniculi penetrate the brainstem to join the solitary nucleus at the bulbopontic junction for the taste fibers and at the spinal nucleus of the trigeminal nerve (V) for the sensory fibers.

The vegetative fibers originate from the lacrimal and superior salivary nuclei, near the motor and solitary nuclei. Some of these fibers become part of the greater petrosal nerve (exiting the petrosal bone at the anterior aspect of the geniculate ganglion), and then, in the pterygoidian nerve to reach the sphenopalatine ganglion. Secretory fibers for the lacrimal gland and the mucosa of the rhinopharynx originate from that point. The other vegetative fibers travel first in the chorda tympani, then the lingual nerve to the submandibular ganglion and give secretory fibers for the submandibular and sublingual glands.

Figure 7.2 and Table 7.1 summarize the distribution and the functions of the different parts constituting the VII nerve.

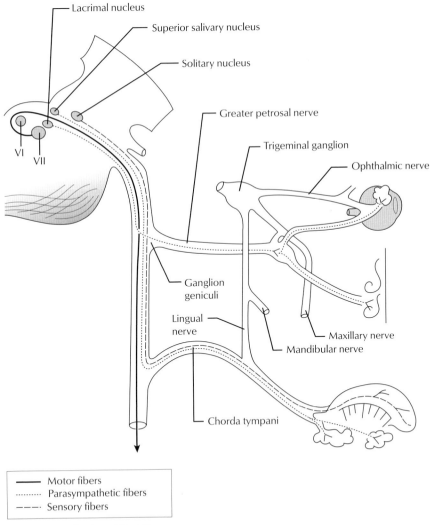

FIGURE 7.2 Systematization of the VII nerve.

TABLE 7.1 Distribution and Functions of the Different Components of the Facial Nerve

Component of the VII Nerve	Distribution
Motor	Stapes, stylohyoid, and posterior belly of digastric muscles; facial platysma and occipital muscles
Sensitive	Conqua of the auricle, the retroauricular area, and (along with the V3), the external acoustic meatus, and the tympanic membrane
Sensory	Taste sensation from the distal two thirds of the tongue and palate
Vegetative	Lacrimal, submandular, and sublingual glands; mucosa of the rhinopharynx and palate

Vascularization

The vascularization of the VII nerve is provided by the anteroinferior cerebellar artery that accompanies the VII nerve in the IAM and through the petrosal branch of the middle meningeal artery and the stylomastoid branch of the retroauricular artery. The territories of these three arteries overlap except in the region of the ganglion geniculi, which may explain why the ganglion geniculi portion is readily exposed to ischemia.

RADIOLOGIC ANATOMY

MR Image

On T2-weighted MR image sequences with inframillimetric sections (three-dimensional fast spin echo [3D-FSE], three-dimensional turbo spin echo [3D-TSE], or constructive interference in steady state [CISS]), the facial nerve can be located in the cerebellopontine trigone in front of the vestibulocochlear nerve, in its anterior concavity. This is readily seen on oblique sagittal sections perpendicular to the IAM. In the IAM, the facial nerve can be found in the anterosuperior quadrant (Fig. 7.3).

In the petrosal pyramid during T1-weighted MRI sequences after gadolinium injection, only the segments that can physiologically take up contrast material (see a frigore facial paralysis, below) can be seen; in some pathologic situations, other segments can be seen.

The facial nerve cannot be isolated in the parotid gland, although the parotid should be studied during the course of a PFP, at least with T1-weighted coronal MRI sections after the injection of contrast material.

Computed Axial Tomography Scanning

High-resolution computed axial tomography (CT) scanning with millimetric sections is used to study of the entire pathway of the facial nerve with direct axial and coronal incidences or with multiple-plane reconstructions from volumetric acquisitions from the axial plane (Fig. 7.4).

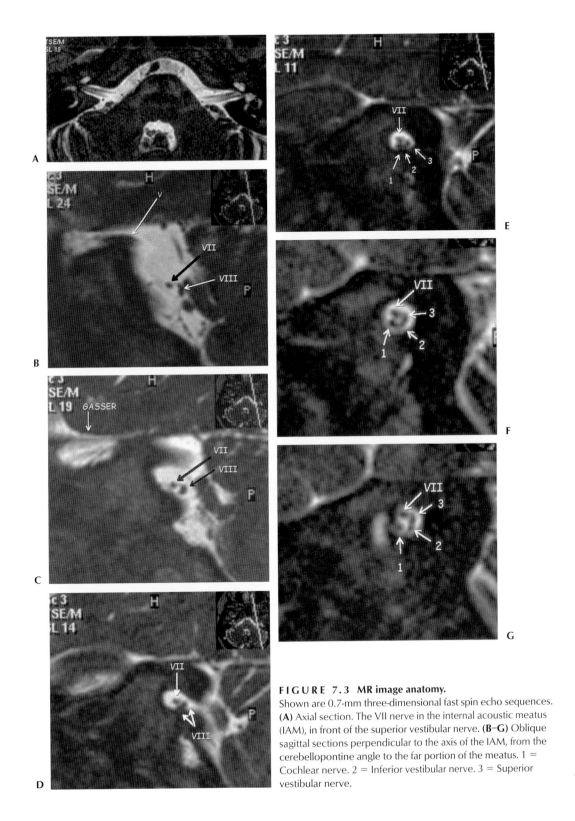

FIGURE 7.3 MR image anatomy.
Shown are 0.7-mm three-dimensional fast spin echo sequences.
(A) Axial section. The VII nerve in the internal acoustic meatus
(IAM), in front of the superior vestibular nerve. **(B–G)** Oblique
sagittal sections perpendicular to the axis of the IAM, from the
cerebellopontine angle to the far portion of the meatus. 1 =
Cochlear nerve. 2 = Inferior vestibular nerve. 3 = Superior
vestibular nerve.

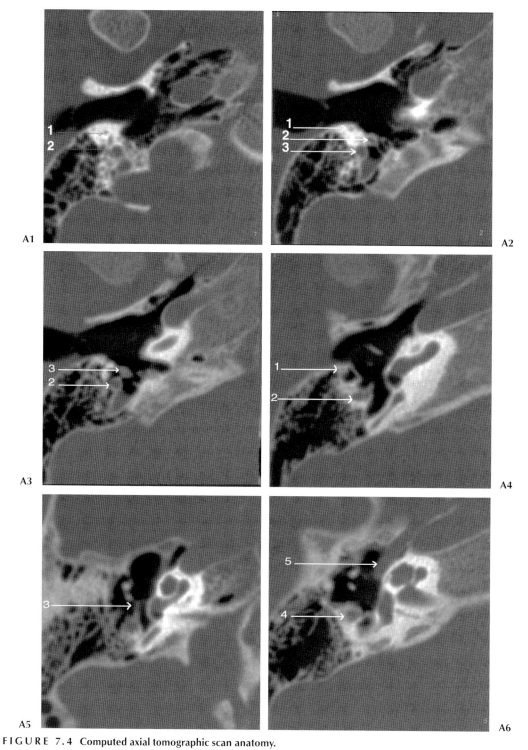

FIGURE 7.4 Computed axial tomographic scan anatomy.
(A) Axial sections 1–9. 1 : Chorda tympani. 2 : The VII nerve. 3 : Tendon of stapes muscle. 4 : Elbow of facial nerve.
5 : Tendon of malleus muscle. 6 : The VII 2 nerve.   *(continues)*

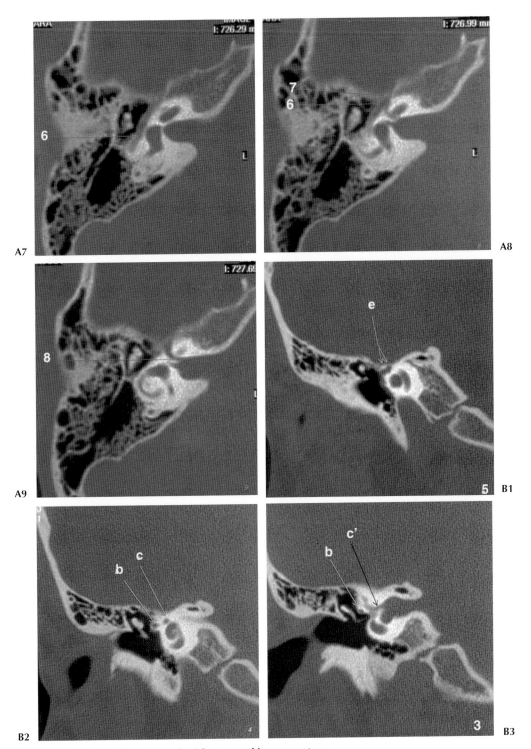

FIGURE 7.4 *(continued)* **Computed axial tomographic scan anatomy.**
(A) 7 : Genu of the facial nerve. 8 : The VII 1 nerve. **(B)** Frontal sections 1–5. a : The VII 3 nerve. b : The VII 2 nerve.
c : The VII 1 nerve. c′ : Superior quadrant of the internal acoustic meatus.   *(continues)*

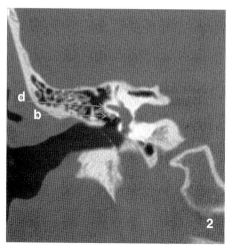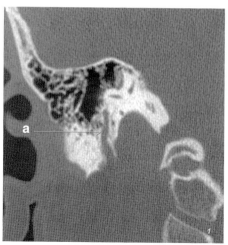

FIGURE 7.4 *(concluded)* **Computed axial tomographic scan anatomy.**
(B) d : Lateral semicircular canal. e : Genu of the facial nerve (behind the ganglion geniculi).

ANATOMIC VARIATIONS/MALPOSITIONS OF THE VII NERVE

Dehiscence of the Canal of the Facial Nerve (Fallopian Aqueduct)

Anatomic variations of the VII nerve are due to the double embryologic origin of the facial nerve's canal: the otic capsule and Reichert cartilage. Ossification of the canal begins at the 10th week of intrauterine life and continues until the end of the first year. The majority of ossification defects are located on the tympanic segment along a 0.5- to 3-mm width. A number of different histologic studies have shown dehiscence in the canal in 55% of cases: 90% were found in the tympanic segment, of which 80% were opposite the vestibular window. Sometimes the nerve herniates through the dehiscence.

During the course of inflammatory disease of the middle ear, dehiscence can increase the risk of facial paralysis.

Anomalies in the Intrapetrous Pathway of the VII Nerve

Malpositions of the VII nerve in the petrosal pyramid can be isolated or, more often, can be associated with malformations of the middle or inner ear. These malpositions should be brought to the attention of the consulting surgeon.

Labyrinthine Portion

The labyrinthic portion of the intrapetrous pathway of the VII nerve can be bifid and can break away in the upper portion of the IAM (Fig. 7.5) or form a completely separate canal from it.

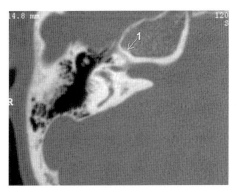

FIGURE 7.5 Pathway anomaly in the labyrinthine portion of the intrapetrous pathway of the VII nerve.
Deafness related to the X chromosome. Axial computed axial tomography scan section: individualization of the VII nerve (1) in the upper portion of the internal acoustic meatus.

Tympanic Portion

The tympanic portion of the intrapetrous pathway of the VII nerve can also be bifid. This portion can be completely absent, particularly in certain severe aplasias, with a very anterior "third" portion. The tympanic portion can also be prominent in front of the vestibular window. In this case, the facial nerve often has a larger diameter and is associated with agenesis of the vestibular window (Fig. 7.6). Finally, the VII nerve can pass entirely or partially between the branches of the stapes. The two last anomalies produce transmission deafness.

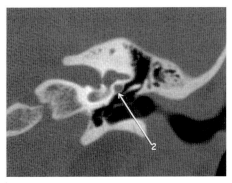

FIGURE 7.6 Left conductive deafness.
Frontal computed axial tomography scan section. VII 2 (2 →) is voluminous and prominent in front of the oval window. Agenesis of the vestibular window.

Mastoid Portion

The mastoid portion of the intrapetrous pathway of the VII nerve can also be bifid. In severe aplasias, the mastoid portion is very often anterior and can travel in the atresic plaque, rendering the creation of a neoconduit (Fig. 7.7) difficult. The mastoid portion can also be absent and the facial nerve can be directed toward the front, near an elbow in the tympanic cavity.

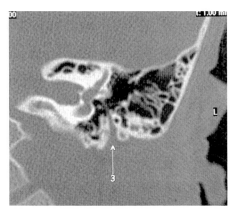

FIGURE 7.7 Aplasia of the left ear.
Frontal section. Absence of an external acoustic meatus. The third portion (3 →) is very anterior and descends directly downward from the vestibular window. The nerve is bare along its route through the tympanic cavity, and further down, the nerve travels along the atresic plaque.

TYPES OF NERVE LESIONS AND FUNCTIONAL TESTS

Functional testing is important in determining the prognosis and is used in the initial workup and the follow-up of facial paralysis. Functional testing techniques can help to quantify the percentage of fibers that are denervated and consequently, allow an assessment of the possibilities for and the quality of recuperation. The pathophysiology of the nerve lesion causing a facial paralysis explains the differences in recuperation as a function of the etiology, duration of the clinical course, and the results of the therapeutic decisions made, partly based on the results of these tests.

Types of Nerve Lesions

The VII nerve is constituted by axons that are isolated from the extracellular spaces by Schwann sheath, which is responsible for demyelinization and furnishes the nerve with oxygen. The axon's cytoplasm, or **axoplasm**, is renewed from its cell body at the rate of 1 mm per day. This corresponds to the axon's regeneration rate after section of the nerve.

Compression or section of the nerve interrupts the regeneration flow of the axoplasm. Sunderland has defined five stages of severity in nerve lesions:

- *Neurapraxia* is the temporary and reversible loss of conduction due to alteration of the myelin sheath, secondary to incomplete compression. Recuperation, which will be complete, begins as early as the 3rd week.

- *Axonotmesis* occurs when the compression is sufficiently important to completely interrupt axoplasmic flow and results in axon death. The supporting sheath is preserved (endoneurium, perineurium, epineurium) and compete recuperation remains possible, albeit more slowly (between 3 weeks and 2 months).

- *Neuronotmesis* is defined by injury to the entire nerve trunk after prolonged compression, with injury to the supporting sheaths. Regeneration requires 2 to 4 months, may be incomplete, and/or may be accompanied by synkinesia (because regrowth of the axon occurs in different directions because to loss of the endoneurium and, consequently, a voluntary movement in a muscle group can produce involuntary and concomitant movement in another territory: eg, untimely blinking of an eye during smiling).

- When **partial** (stage 4) or **complete** (stage 5) nerve section occurs, spontaneous recuperation is impossible and appropriate surgery is required.

In the majority of idiopathic and herpetic facial paralysis cases, nerve injury is limited to the first two stages. Stages 4 and 5 are seen in facial paralysis due to tumor or trauma. Prolonged compression or added vascular phenomena can worsen the stage; hence the importance of functional testing to consider early surgical decompression.

Functional Testing and Assessment of Severity

The facial nerve contains approximately 7,000 myelinated fibers. Functional testing allows a quantification of the proportion of degenerated fibers compared with the uninvolved side. This permits an assessment of the possibilities for motor recovery and for anticipating complications (facial hemispasm, synkinesia). Functional testing is also useful in the recovery phase. However, functional tests are of little use when facial paralysis is incomplete and are useless when the patient has a history of contralateral facial paralysis.

Electroneuronography or Esslen Test

Electroneuronography (ENG) is undoubtedly the best test; it is both objective and quantitative. ENG results provide definite prognostic information and ENG should be performed around the 10th day. Skin surface electrodes are used to gather the composite muscular action potential (CMAP) at the nasolabial angle after stimulation of the nerve at the level of the stylomastoid foramen. The spike-to-spike CMAP amplitude is proportional to the number of degenerated fibers and can be compared with the unaffected side. Normally, the difference between the 2 sides is less than 3%. During PFP, if the percentage of degenerated fibers is greater than 90%, less than 50% of the patients will have good recuperation. ENG testing can also be performed in infants.

Hilger Test or Minimal Nerve Excitability Test

The Hilger test uses stimulation of the nerve at the stylomastoid orifice to determine the lowest electrical threshold needed to obtain a visible facial contraction on the affected and unaffected sides. A greater than 3.5-mA difference between the two sides constitutes an unfavorable result. The Hilger test is subjective and should be performed before the 10th day and should be repeated by the same examiner.

Electromyography

Electromyography (EMG) consists of recording muscular activity by pricking the different muscle groups of the face with a needle. Spontaneous electrical activity (fibrillation) must be differentiated from voluntary electrical activity. During the course of severe facial paralysis, spontaneous discharges in the denervated muscles, called fibrillation potentials, can be seen but only appear a few days after onset. The presence of significant spontaneous activity indicates marked denervation and suggests poorer chances for recovery. Inversely, the persistence of potentials in motor units during voluntary contractions is a good prognostic sign.

PERIPHERAL FACIAL PARALYSIS

Clinical Presentation

Complete peripheral facial paralysis produces facial asymmetry to the point of making the diagnosis very obvious: at rest, the paralyzed side is smooth with disappearance of wrinkles, the mouth is deviated toward the unaffected side, and the eye opening is widened. This asymmetry is intensified by both voluntary and spontaneous facial grimaces. The Bell sign consists of the inability to close the eyelids on the paralyzed side, with upward deviation of the eye beneath the upper eyelid. Traction on the tongue causes it to deviate toward the unaffected side because of the deformation of the paralyzed commissura laborium.

Facial paralysis can be minimal, necessitating a meticulous examination to discover clinical signs that predominate at the eyelids (Souques sign: the eyelids appear to be longer on the paralyzed side when the eyelids are closed, with asymmetric blinking). The comatose patient's flaccid cheek fills with each expiration and the patient's grimace is asymmetric when provoked by a painful stimulus.

The clinical examination should try to exclude central facial paralysis, which spares the superior facial territory with conservation of spontaneous reflex motor activity. Most often, central facial paralysis is accompanied by other neurologic deficits (hemiplegia or brachial monoplegia). During the initial physical examination, PFP should be quantified by comparative testing of motor activity in the 10 muscle groups (rated from 0 to 5) and for muscle tone (rated 0 to 3). These assessments should be repeated by the same examiner during follow-up examinations to determine if there is improvement. The classification by House and Brackmann, which assesses both muscle strength and tone, is the one most often used (Table 7.2).

Etiologic Diagnosis

The patient history and the results of the physical examination are often useful for orienting the etiologic diagnosis:

- Presence of vertigo, tinnitus, deafness, painful hyperacousia, disorders of taste
- History of trauma, a vesicular skin rash in the Ramsay-Hunt area, a middle ear infection, a parotid mass, or an associated paralysis in another cranial nerve

Additional studies can also help reduce the etiologic possibilities:

- Systematic studies: Tonal audiometry, a vestibular examination, otoscopic examination.
- Localizing procedures: The Schirmer test, the stapes reflex, and gustometry. The Schirmer test compares lacrimal secretions on the paralyzed and unaffected side; when the results of the Schirmer test are abnormal, it is indicative that the lesion is proximal to the origin of the greater petrosal nerve or along its pathway.
- The stapes reflex disappears when the lesion is proximal to the origin of the nerve supplying the stapes muscle, but this reflex is dependent on the integrity of the entire reflex arc: eg, eardrum, ossicular chain, cochlea.
- Gustometry is abnormal when the lesion is proximal to the starting point of the chorda tympani.
- Functional testing (see above) provides valuable prognostic information.
- Imaging is important in the etiologic diagnosis and in the workup for localizing the lesion; when performed, imaging modalities should study the entire pathway of the VII nerve. CT scanning or MRI should be the first procedures performed according to the suspected etiology.

Table 7.3 summarizes the clinical aspects, the results of other diagnostic procedures, and the different lesions with respect to the affected segment.

TABLE 7.2 Quantification of PFP by Using House and Brackmann's Classification.

Grade/Description	Facial Function	Symmetry and Muscle Tone at Rest	Symptoms and Signs
Grade 1: Normal	Normal facial function		
Grade II: Slight injury	Slight weakness noticeable on examination	Normal symmetry and muscle tone	Movements: forehead: normal; eye: normal closure, slight asymmetry; lips: movements slightly asymmetric **Hemispasm, contractures, synkinesia:** absent.
Grade III: Moderate injury	Identical on both sides, no facial distortion	Normal symmetry and muscle tone	Movements: forehead: slight or absent; eye: closure with effort, asymmetry; lips: movement very asymmetric **Hemispasm, contractures, synkinesia:** severe
Grade IV: Moderately severe injury	Obvious weakness and/or asymmetry without facial distortion	Normal symmetry and muscle tone	Movements: forehead: absent; eye: complete closure impossible; lips: asymmetric movement during effort **Hemispasm, contractures, synkinesia:** absent
Grade V: Severe injury	Movement: very attenuated	Asymmetry possible	Movements: forehead: absent; eye: incomplete closure, slight movement of eyelids; lips: attenuated movements **Hemispasm, contractures, synkinesia:** absent
Grade VI: Total paralysis	Total paralysis	Loss of both tone and symmetry	Movements: all impossible **Hemispasm, contractures,** synkinesia: absent

TABLE 7.3 Topographic Diagnosis of Lesions to the Facial Nerve: Choice of Imaging Procedure (IP)

Segment	Clinical Aspect/Tests	IP	Lesions
Nuclear: Pons	VII + VII	MRI	Infarction, hematoma, multiple sclerosis, tumor, arteriovenous malformation, cavernous angioma, abscess
CPA + IAM	VII + VIII; audiometry: perception deafness, vestibular examination	MRI	Neurinoma of VIII nerve, meningioma, epidermoid cyst, vascular compression, neurinoma of the VII nerve, hemangioma, glomus tumor, inflammation, fracture
Ganglion geniculi	Schirmer test	CT scan or MRI	Neurinoma and hemangioma of VII nerve, primary of secondary cholesteatoma, cholesterol granuloma, metastasis, infection, fracture
Tympanic membrane or mastoid	Audiometry: transmission deafness, otoscopic examination, stapes reflex, gustometry	CT scan	Acute otitis, mastoiditis, cholesteatoma, fracture, neurinoma of VII nerve, necrotic otitis externa, metastasis, glomus tumor
Parotid and endings	Often partial involvement	MRI	Often malignant parotid tumor, infection, sarcoidosis, trauma (forceps, penetrating lesion, surgery)

CT, computed axial tomography; MRI, MR image.

Imaging Techniques

A complete MRI study is necessary to determine the etiologic diagnosis. MRI studies should include the following sequences:

- A T2-weighted sequence of the entire skull so that an inflammatory process, a demyelinating disorder (Fig. 7.8), or multiple tumors are not overlooked.

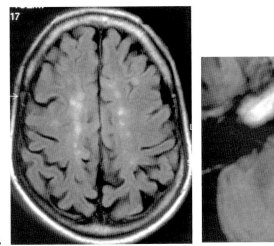 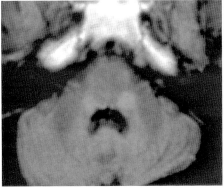

A   B

FIGURE 7.8 Multiple sclerosis.
Left facial paralysis. Fluid-attenuated inversion recovery MR image sequence, axial sections. **(A)** Through the pons.
Bilateral hypersignals at the anterior surface of V4. **(B)** Supratentorial section. Bilateral periventricular hypersignals.

- A 3D-TSE or CISS T2-weighted sequence using an axial incidence with millimetric sections to study the VII nerve in the cerebellopontine angle (CPA) and the IAM.
- A T1-weighted sequence before the injection of contrast material, using an axial incidence.
- Two T1-weighted sequences after the injection of contrast material, using axial and coronal incidences, with the coronal section important in studying the parotid gland.
- To unfold the second and third portions, a sagittal incidence may be helpful (Fig. 7.9).

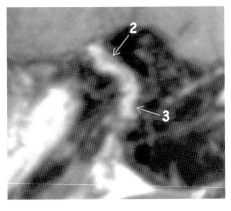

FIGURE 7.9 Right neurinoma of the III nerve.
T1-weighted oblique sagittal MR image section after contrast injection. Thickening of the 2nd (2 →) and 3rd (3 →) portions with enhancement and clear marking of the pathway of the VII nerve.

- High-resolution MRI (HR-MRI) should be ordered immediately after traumatic injury when complications during the course of an inflammatory process of the middle ear are suspected, for assessing malformations, and in conjunction with standard MRI when bone spread from a tumor is suspected. Axial and directed coronal incidences should be performed or reconstructed after spiral axial acquisition. In spiral axial acquisition, inframillimetric sections are preferable, notably for studying the tympanic segment (whose shell can be dehiscent or can be in an opaque cavity).

Differential Diagnosis of PFP in Adults

At the end of this chapter, a decision tree (DT 1) is given as a function of the clinical presentation; the topographic localization of the lesion is equally important and relies on the associated clinical signs and other localizing procedures (Table 7.3).

Idiopathic Facial Paralysis or Bell's Palsy

This is the most frequent cause of PFP (60% of the cases in a series of 1500) and is probably due to herpes simplex virus (HSV 1). Typically, it has a sudden, unilateral onset that is often preceded by a viral prodrome. Most often, Bell palsy spontaneously regresses in 8 to 10 weeks.

Imaging should only be considered in atypical cases: eg, bilateral involvement, no regression or only partial regression, ipsilateral recurrent PFP, other focal neurologic signs.

MRI with contrast injection shows intense contrast uptake by the paralyzed nerve from the far end of the IAM to the mastoid segment. This enhancement should be distinguished from the physiologic uptake of the nerve, which predominates along the ganglion geniculi and the tympanic segment, is often not very intense, and never involves the far end of the IAM or the labyrinthine segment. The intensity of the enhancement has no prognostic value and can persist for a number of weeks after resolution of the PFP. Contrast uptake should be linear; in cases of a nodular appearance, a tumor should be suspected. A recent study demonstrated that with 3D-FSE T2 sequences using inframillimetric sections and reconstructions perpendicular and parallel to the VII nerve in the meatus, there was localized thickening in the nerve in the far end of the IAM in 21 of 22 patients in the series who had herpetic or idiopathic PFP. This enhancement, which was visible with high resolution, could not be seen on the T1 sequence after contrast injection, with the intensity of the enhancement preventing clear delimitation of the nerve's borders.

Posttraumatic Facial Paralysis

Most often, traumatic lesions to the facial nerve occur in its intrapetrous portion. Nevertheless, traumatic lesions along the brainstem, the CPA, or in the parotid also occur. Petrosal bone fractures are accompanied by PFP in 20% of longitudinal, extralabyrinthine fractures and in 30 to 50% of transversal fractures, most of which are translabyrinthine. CT scanning is the most effective imaging procedure for studying fracture lines and ossicular displacement or for studying an eventual bone impaction (Figure 7.10). MRI can detect dissecting hematomas of the nerve and can thus guide decompression when surgery is indicated.

In longitudinal fractures, most often the nerve is injured around the ganglion geniculi and the onset of paralysis is differed and is often incomplete and regressive. In transversal fractures, PFP is often sudden and complete and due to transection or laceration of the nerve by bone splinters. The nerve can be injured along its entire intrapetrous pathway; when functional testing demonstrates complete degeneration, early surgery (during the 1st week) may be indicated.

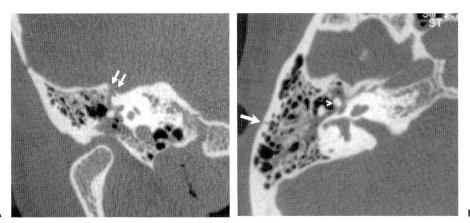

A   B

FIGURE 7.10 Longitudinal fracture of the petrosal bone. Immediate-onset facial paralysis.
(A) Axial section. The fracture line passes through the mastoid (→) and extends toward the anterior attic. Bone dislocation and impaction of the head of the malleus (➤) along its second portion are seen. (B) Coronal section. Fracture line in the tegmen also passing through the second portion (→→).

The Special Case of Postoperative PFP

During surgery for lesions in the CPA or the IAM, the risk of facial paralysis increases with the size of the lesion; the surgeon can monitor the nerve during the intervention. In middle ear surgery, this risk is higher in ears that have undergone surgical treatment multiple times and also in ears with malformations; in both cases, anatomic landmarks are usually disrupted. Finally, in parotid gland surgery, risk is greatest when the deep lobe is involved. Imaging is required when injury to the nerve was not apparent during surgery or when impairment cannot be explained by surgery that has been performed in the immediate area.

Infectious Disorders

Ramsay-Hunt Syndrome. Ramsay-Hunt syndrome is the third most frequent cause of PFP, after idiopathic and posttraumatic PFP. It is caused by **Herpes zoster oticus** and the symptoms are more severe than in idiopathic facial paralysis, often including dizziness, perception deafness (due to involvement of the vestibulocochlear nerve), and intense otalgia. A vesicular skin lesion in the Ramsay-Hunt area confirms the diagnosis. During MRI, there is contrast uptake that often affects all of the nerves in the IAM and sometimes the labyrinth. It can occasionally be difficult to differentiate Ramsay-Hunt syndrome from a schwannoma (Fig. 7.11).

     Inflammatory Lesions of the Middle Ear. Acute otitis media can be responsible for a PFP that usually regresses after antibiotic treatment or myringotomy. CT scanning can demonstrate dehiscence of the tympanic segment, a predisposing factor for this complication.

     In chronic otitis, regardless of whether it is complicated by a cholesteatoma, facial paralysis indicates compression of the nerve by the cholesteatoma or osteitis. Immediately before surgery, CT scanning can show the site of the compression by demonstrating destruction of the walls of the facial canal and the causal lesion.

     Necrotic Otitis Externa. Necrotic otitis externa is due to *Pseudomonas aeruginosa* infection and occurs in elderly diabetic patients. The VII nerve is invaded through the stylomastoid foramen. This disorder is difficult to differentiate from malignant tumors.

     Other Infectious Causes. Lyme disease is complicated by facial paralysis in 10% of cases; paralysis is bilateral in 25% of cases and can be the initial symptom of the disease. MRI shows

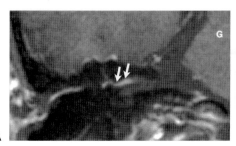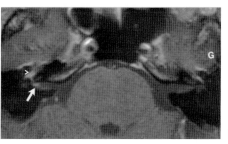

A   B

FIGURE 7.11   Right idiopathic peripheral facial paralysis.
T1-weighted axial (**A**) and frontal (**B**) IRM sections following contrast injection. Enhancement of the VII nerve at the far end of the internal acoustic meatus (→), of the labyrinthine portion, and of the ganglion geniculi (➤). The right ganglion geniculi are slightly more voluminous than the left. This can also suggest a schwannoma.

nonspecific contrast uptake in the nerve but there is often disseminated neuritis with enhancement in a number of different cranial nerves in the absence of any clinical correlation.

Involvement of the VII nerve during the course of acquired immunodeficiency syndrome is also nonspecific. Consequently, systematic supratentorial studies, at least in T2, can be useful.

Tumors

Progressive PFP with a slow onset of more than 3 weeks should indicate a tumor etiology despite the fact that tumors can also produce sudden onset or relapsing facial paralysis.

In the brainstem, primary or secondary tumors produce impairment in a number of cranial nerve pairs.

In the cerebellopontine angle and the internal acoustic meatus, the most frequent lesions in the CPA and IAM are **neurinomas of the VIII nerve** and **meningiomas.** During MRI, neurinomas, which are described in chapter 8 (p. 163), are often easy to distinguish from meningiomas because of their wide base of implantation, which is excentrically located with respect to the porus of the IAM, and because of their intense and homogeneous contrast uptake.

Epidermoid cysts have a signal similar to that of cerebrospinal fluid (CSF) in T1 and T2 sequences, although epidermoid cysts are slightly more hyperintense. They have irregular contours and can spread supratentorially through the Pacchioni foramen.

Arachnoid cysts are isointense with respect to CSF, have sharp contours, and remain confined to the subtentorial space. These cysts produce a frank mass effect on adjacent structures (brainstem, cerebellum, acoustic–facial packet, bone) (Fig. 7.12). Nevertheless, arachnoid and epidermoid cysts can be difficult to distinguish from one another and from surrounding CSF. Fluid-attenuated inversion recovery MRI sequences (suppression of the signal coming from the CSF) can help detect epidermoid cysts; diffusion sequences show reduced diffusion within an epidermoid cyst compared with an arachnoid cyst.

In the internal acoustic meatus and the region of the ganglion geniculi, during CT scan, **neurinomas of the VII nerve** are manifested by regular widening of the IAM and/or the facial canal. The nerve appears enlarged during MRI with homogeneous contrast uptake and when they spread to the tympanic and mastoid portions, neurinomas clearly delineate the intrapetrous pathway of the VII nerve (Fig. 7.9). Neurinomas can also develop from the ganglion geniculi toward the middle temporal fossa. Although neurinomas can be very large, they do not always produce facial paralysis. In contrast, **hemangiomas** are small lesions that are associated with notable clinical manifestations: perception deafness, rigidity, or facial paresis. CT scanning demonstrates irregular bone

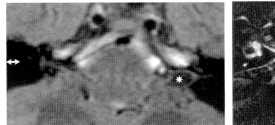
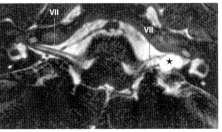

FIGURE 7.12 Arachnoid cyst of the left internal acoustic meatus (IAM).
Left anacousia . Facial paralysis. Axial three-dimensional fast spin echo MR image section. On the left, the distance between the VII (→) and the VIII nerves in the cerebellopontine angle is increased, the VII nerve is distorted and pushed toward the front by the cyst (★), which has sharp contours and widens the IAM. Axial T2 fluid-attenuated inversion recovery MRI section. The cyst (★) is isointense with respect to cerebrospinal fluid.

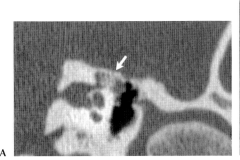
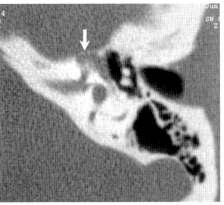

FIGURE 7.13 Hemangioma of the right VII nerve.
(A) Computed axial tomography scan, axial section. Widening of the labyrinthine portion and of the fossula of the ganglion geniculi by a mass containing delicate calcifications (→). (B) Frontal reconstruction. Identical aspect and distortion of the roof of the petrosal bone (→). Films reproduced courtesy of Dr. Marc Williams (Rothschild Foundation).

erosion and delicate "beehive" calcifications (Fig. 7.13). These lesions are often hyperintense during T1 and T2 MRI, with areas containing no signal, probably corresponding to **flow-void** areas (high-flow blood vessels) or to calcifications.

In the tympanic cavity and the mastoid, otoscopic examination can suggest tumor in the tympanic cavity and the mastoid by showing a whitish (**primary cholesteatoma**), grayish (*i*), or bluish (**glomus**) retrotympanic mass. Primary cholesteatomas and **cholesterol granulomas** can be differentiated by their T1 appearance: cholesterol granulomas are hyperintense because of the accumulation of blood degradation products. The **jugulotympanic glomus** is accompanied by bone destruction, intense contrast uptake in both CT scan and MRI, and empty signal areas during MRI, related to high-flow areas. Finally, primary or secondary bone tumors can be seen in the petrosal bone.

In the parotid gland, every parotid mass associated with facial paralysis should suggest a malignancy. The use of a surface antenna during MRI can improve spatial resolution. Sequences with fat suppressed cancel out the spinal cord fat at the base of the skull as well as subcutaneous fat, resulting in better delineation of contrast uptake. Perineural diffusion should be sought for by following the VII nerve along its third portion; **cystic adenoid carcinomas** or **cylindromas** can frequently be discovered.

The **peripheral branches** cannot be directly studied; however, their target organs can be studied. The peripheral branches can contain tumors that have spread by the perineural route.

Clinical Forms

Facial paralysis can be bilateral:

- Sarcoidosis: Facial diplegia and uveitis.
- Guillain-Barré syndrome: Facial diplegia, velopharyngeal involvement, and impairment in the sensory and motor nerves of the extremities.
- Lyme disease (see above).
- Leukosis: Identical MRI findings in the VII nerve as seen in idiopathic PFP. An associated parenchymal or meningeal lesion should be searched for; hence the importance of studying the supratentorial level.
- Recurrent clinical forms: Melkersson-Rosenthal syndrome associated with alternate-side, recurrent PFP, lip edema, and increased tongue folds. MRI shows the same enhancement as that seen in idiopathic PFP.

The Differential Diagnosis of Peripheral Facial Nerve (PFNP) Paralysis in Infants

A decision-tree (DT 2) as a function of the clinical presentation is shown at the end of this chapter.

Neonatal Facial Paralysis

Obstetric Facial Paralysis. At birth, the mastoid is still poorly developed and the third portion of the facial canal, which is superficial, is exposed to trauma by crushing and fracture, most often related to the use of forceps, but injury can also be seen after spontaneous delivery or may be caused by a pathologic intrauterine position. The resulting facial paralysis spontaneously regresses in a couple of weeks. CT scanning is indicated when there is no regression after 2 months to exclude a dish-pan fracture that requires early surgical decompression (before age 3 months) to be efficacious.

Facial Paralysis Due to Malformations. *Isolated Hypoplasia of the VII Nerve.* High-resolution CT scan shows a reduction in the caliber of the facial canal, reflecting hypoplasia of the nerve on the paralyzed side (Fig. 7.14).

Moebius Syndrome. Typically, Moebius syndrome is associated with facial diplegia and paralysis of the abducens nerves, but there are unilateral forms associated with impairment in other ipsilateral cranial nerves. Moebius syndrome is probably caused by antenatal ischemia of the nuclei of the nerves in the brainstem. MRI shows brainstem hypoplasia and no nerves in the cerebellopontine trigone.

Hypoplasia of the Ear. Often, malposition of the VII nerve is seen with hypoplasia of the ear (see Fig. 7.6), but facial paralysis is less commonly observed.

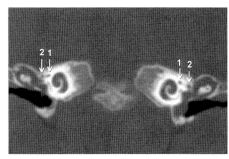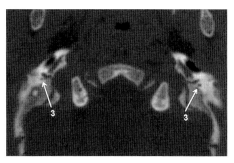

FIGURE 7.14 Hypoplasia of the right VII nerve.
(**A**) Computed axial tomography (CT) scan, frontal section. Clear asymmetry of the first (1→) and second (2→) portions of the fallopian aqueduct; the diameter on the right is smaller. (**B**) CT scan, axial section. Smaller diameter on the third portion (→) on the right.

Facial Paralysis in Infants

A frigore facial paralysis is less commonly seen in infants than in adults but remains the more frequent etiology (40–60% of cases). The recuperation rate for a frigore facial paralysis in infants is higher than in adults.

Some other elements particular to infants include the following:

1. Posttraumatic PFP is frequent.
2. The **frequency of PFP after otitis** (acute otitis media, mastoiditis, cholesteatoma) is as high as 25% in some series.
3. **Other infectious causes:** Enterovirus (poliovirus, echovirus), herpes virus (herpes zoster, Epstein-Barr virus), mumps, Lyme disease, suppurating meningitis. These infectious agents are sometimes responsible for facial diplegias.
4. **PFP caused by tumor:**
   A. In the brainstem: Glioma
   B. In the CPA: Neurinomas are rare but can occur during the course of type 2 neurofibromatosis, which, as a general rule, does not appear before the second decade of life (Fig. 7.15)
   C. In the petrosal pyramid: Rhabdomyosarcoma
5. Other diseases:
   A. Blood diseases: Leukosis, lymphomas
   B. Systemic: Langherans histiocytosis
   C. Bone diseases: Osteopetrosis (Fig. 7.16), idiopathic hypercalcemia

HEMIFACIAL SPASM

Hemifacial spasm is characterized by in the sudden, painless, involuntary contraction of the muscles innervated by the VII nerve. Hemifacial spasm is most often due to a conflict between vascular structures and the nerve at the **root exit zone** (REZ), which is an approximately 3-mm area beginning at the emergence of the VII nerve from the brainstem, at the junction of the central-type and peripheral-type myelin fibers.

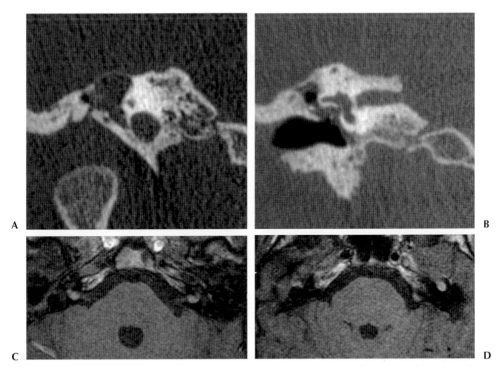

A

B

C

D

FIGURE 7.15 Type 2 neurofibromatosis in a 15-year-old boy. Chronic otitis. Right peripheral facial paralysis for 1 year.
(A) CT scan, frontal section. Mass located in the anterior attic eroding the fossula of the ganglion geniculi and raising the tegmen. **(B)** CT scan, frontal section through the vestibular window. Hypopneumatization and condensation in the mastoid, retraction of the tympanic membrane. Filling of the cavity; the bony coccus of the 2nd portion is not visible. **(C)** MRI, axial section after injection of contrast material passing through the internal acoustic meatus. Bilateral contrast uptake in the canal. **(D)** MR image, axial section through the ganglion geniculi after injection of contrast material . Bilateral nodular contrast uptake, which is more voluminous on the right.

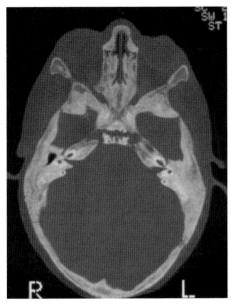

FIGURE 7.16 Osteopetrosis.
Computed axial tomography scan, axial section. The base of the skull is dense and the mastoids and the ethmoid are filled. The VII nerve may be injured along its labyrinthine portion (stenosis of the foramen of the base) and in the mastoid.

The vascular structures involved are, by decreasing order of frequency, the posteroinferior cerebellar artery, the vertebral artery, the anteroinferior cerebellar artery, and a vein (respectively 67%, 52%, 25%, 11% in Magnan's series of 183 patients).

MRI studies should include a high-resolution (CISS, 3D-FSE) T2-weighted sequence capable of clearly defining the vascular-to-nerve relationships, MR angiography with native section analysis and reconstructions. Supratentorial T2 sequences and T1 sequences after the injection of contrast material are also indispensable for excluding a demyelinating or intra-axial disorder or a tumor along the pathway of the VII nerve to the parotid gland.

A vascular structure can be considered responsible for the symptoms when it is in contact with the REZ, is perpendicular to the nerve, and distorts the nerve and/or brainstem (Fig. 7.17).

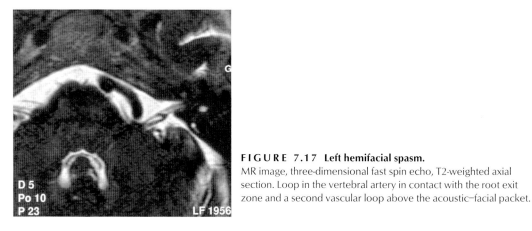

FIGURE 7.17 Left hemifacial spasm.
MR image, three-dimensional fast spin echo, T2-weighted axial section. Loop in the vertebral artery in contact with the root exit zone and a second vascular loop above the acoustic–facial packet.

DT 1: PERIPHERAL FACIAL PARALYSIS IN ADULTS: DIAGNOSTIC WORK-UP

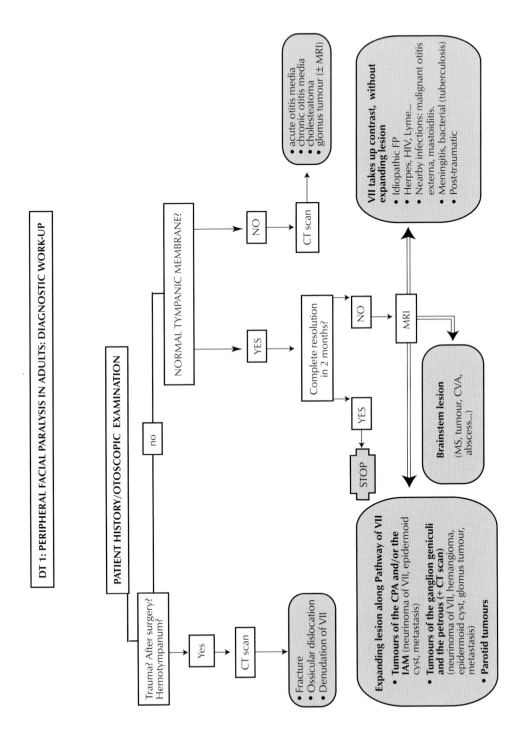

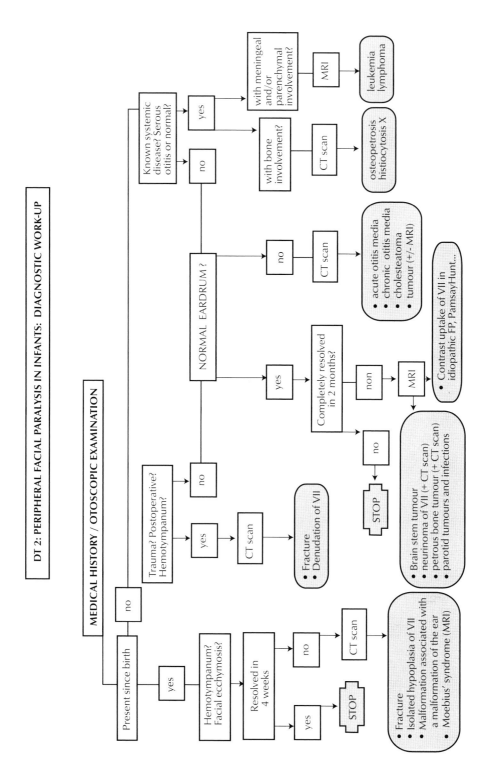

DT 2: PERIPHERAL FACIAL PARALYSIS IN INFANTS: DIAGNOSTIC WORK-UP

MEDICAL HISTORY / OTOSCOPIC EXAMINATION

CHAPTER 8

Vestibulocochlear Nerve (VIII)

K. Marsot-Dupuch and M. Gayet-Delacroix

The origin of perception deafness, disorders of equilibrium, or tinnitus can be located at any point on the sound perception axis or the equilibrium system. Diagnostic studies are used to guide imaging to limit cost. Tonal audiometry and auditory evoked potentials (AEP) of the brainstem can help differentiate endo- and retrocochlear perception deafness but there is a nonnegligible number of false negatives. The electronystagmogram (ENG) tests the reactivity of the vestibule to different temperatures. The result is pathologic when there is a 30% difference in response between the curves of the two vestibules. Functional auditory MR imaging is one of the more promising ways of research for exploring the auditory tract. Its development has provided encouraging results, especially in preoperative workups before cochlear implants and for tinnitus.

TOPOGRAPHIC AND FUNCTIONAL ANATOMY

Auditory Tract

Sensory Organ

The cochlea is part of the anterior labyrinth and is constituted by a hollow tube coiled around itself for two and one-half turns. The lamina spiralis ossea isolates two noncommunicating compartments with different structures: one, the cochlear conduit, is filled with endolymph and contains endocellular-type fluid, whereas the other contains perilymph and contains extracellular-type fluid. The perilymphatic structure limits two levels, the vestibular ramp above and the tympanic ramp below (Fig. 8.1). The perilymphatic compartment communicates with the window of the vestibule (oval) through the vestibular ramp. The tympanic ramp communicates with the window of the cochlea (round). These two ramps communicate with one another through a small channel, the helicotrema, which is located at the apex of the cochlea (Fig. 8.2).

Sound perception is accomplished by the transmission of mechanical vibrations from the sound source to the inner ear. The vibrations are amplified in the middle ear by the ossicula system and by the small surface of the vestibular window.

The liquid vibrations induced by movement in the stapes are transmitted to the vestibular window. From there, the vibrations are transmitted to the perilymph, then to the ciliated cells of the Corti spiral organ (basal lamina), and finally to the cochlear nerve. The apex of the cochlea codes low frequencies, whereas high frequencies are coded by the basal tower. The subarachnoid and endolymphatic spaces can communicate through the modiolus, the pathway taken by the cochlear nerve. The labyrinth has a terminal-type vascularization and is consequently very vulnerable to ischemia.

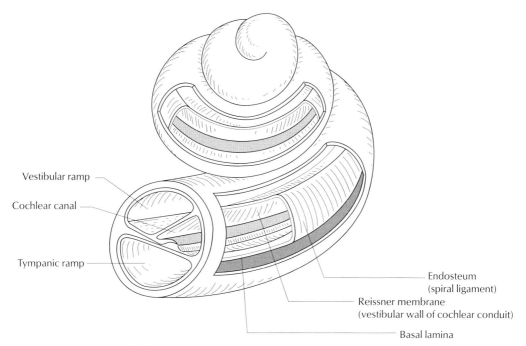

FIGURE 8.1 Anatomy of the inner ear.
The three ramps of the inner ear: the vestibular ramp above, the tympanic ramp below, and the endocochlear canal separated by the Reissner membrane.

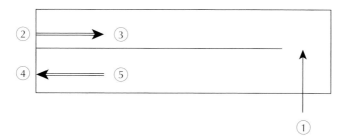

FIGURE 8.2 Transmission of wave sounds to the sensory cells.
1 : Helicotrema. 2 : Vestibular window (oval). 3 : Vestibular ramp. 4 : Window of the cochlea (round). 5 : Vestibular ramp.

Nerve

The cochlear nerve is formed near the modiolus and travels in the internal acoustic meatus (IAM) in its anteroinferior compartment, below the facial nerve and in front of the utricular (superior vestibular) and saccular (inferior vestibular) nerves (Fig. 8.3). After traveling through the CPA, the nerve penetrates into the brainstem up to the ventral and dorsal cochlear nuclei located opposite the inferior cerebellar peduncle. At the level of the pons (level of the cochlear nuclei), the auditory tract crosses the midline near the trapezoid body and climbs back to the lateral lemniscus up to the inferior colliculus (caudal). It attains the medial genicula body and from there, reaches (at the level of the cerebral peduncles) the auditory cortex (transversal temporal gyrus (Fig. 8.4).

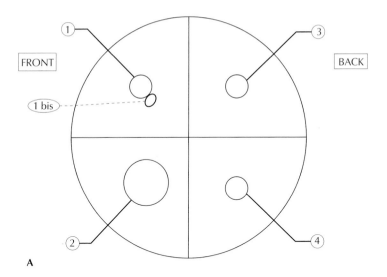

A

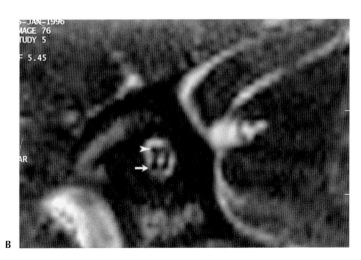

B

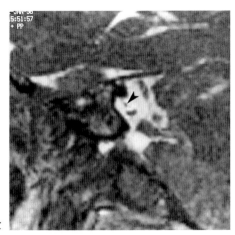

C

FIGURE 8.3 Profile view of the internal acoustic meatus.
(A) In front, the cochlear nerve (2), the most voluminous, is beneath the facial (1) and the intermediate (1 bis) nerves (which are actually impossible to differentiate) and in front of the cephalad utricular (3) and the caudate saccular (4) nerves.
(B) Sagittal section through the acoustic–facial packet: presence of four nodules with an intermediate signal: in front, the facial nerve (➤); behind, the superior vestibular utricular nerve; below and in front, the cochlear nerve (→); and below and behind, the saccular nerve (inferior vestibular). **(C)** Sagittal midline section passing through the cerebellopontine angle. The acoustic–vestibular bundle is indissociable, and the facial nerve is cephalad (➤).

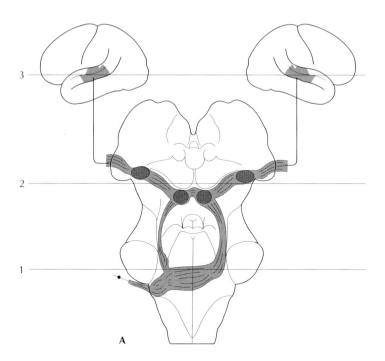

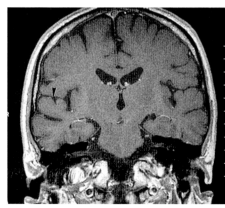

FIGURE 8.4 The auditory pathway.
(A) Sound transmission from the cerebellopontine angle to the
cerebral cortex. Section through the superior and inferior
cochlear nuclei opposite the inferior cerebellar peduncle (plane
1). Decussation near the pons at the level of the trapezoid body
(plane 2). Pathway in the lateral lemniscus to the caudal
colliculus and the medial geniculate body followed by the
auditory cortex (superior temporal gyrus) (plane 3). **(B)** T1-
weighted coronal section through the auditory pathways after
gadolinium injection . Superior temporal gyrus (➤).

Vestibular Pathways

Sensory Cells

The vestibule detects accelerations of linear movement thanks to the ampullae of the semicircular
canals, which contain receptors sensitive to angular displacements.

Vestibular Nerve Fibers

Vestibular nerve fibers pass through the perforated spaces or cribriform spots, forming the utricular and saccular nerves. The posterior ampullar nerve penetrates into the IAM by a separate canal
(**Morgagni's foramen singulare**).

The vestibular nerve fibers travel along the posterior portion of the IAM, then the vestibular nerve penetrates into the brainstem to reach the vestibular nuclei, located in the floor of the IVth ventricle. Connections exist between the vestibular, visual, and cerebellar tracts.

Nonsensory Parts of the Inner Ear

Nonsensory parts of the inner ear consist of the aqueducts of the cochlea and the vestibule (endolymphatic duct and sac), whose function is to equilibrate pressure and to assist ion exchanges between the fluids contained in the peri- and endolymphatic compartments.

Aqueduct of the Vestibule

The aqueduct of the vestibule contains the fluid-filled endolymphatic sac and conduit. The endolymphatic conduit originates at the utricular and saccular conduits, bends at a right angle, and joins the endolymphatic sac at the superior and lateral portion of the endocranial, posterior surface of the petrosal. The endolymphatic sac and duct play a role in the secretion and the absorption of the endolymphatic fluid and in the inner ear's immune defenses. The aqueduct of the vestibule is extradural and mostly extraosseous, and is proximal to the lateral sinus, which it can surround (Fig. 8.5). The small quantity of fluid and the relative thickness of its walls explain why its T1/T2 signal is different from the signal coming from the labyrinth's fluids. During MRI, it can be seen in axial and sagittal sections.

Aqueduct of the Cochlea

The aqueduct of the cochlea is a partially obliterated canal, which presents a double obliquity downward and medially, uniting the basal turn of the cochlea to the jugular foramen (Fig. 8.5). The aqueduct of the cochlea constitutes a potential communication between the subarachnoid and perilymphatic spaces.

IMAGING

MRI is the first procedure to be performed; computed axial tomography scanning is used to study the bony labyrinth and the base of the skull.

MR Image

MRI sequences should involve the different anatomic structures of the auditory and vestibular pathways and should study the connections between the sensory organ and the brainstem as well as their brain relays.

Labyrinth and the Internal Acoustic Meatus

T1-Weighted Sequence Without Gadolinium Injection. Normally, the labyrinthine fluids radiate an intermediate signal resembling cerebrospinal fluid. A T1-weighted MRI sequence without gadolinium injection can document the presence of a spontaneous signal anomaly in the labyrinthine fluids and the CPA (Table 8.1). Spontaneous labyrinthine hypersignals are seen in hemorrhages, lipomas, and in certain calcifications (Fig. 8.6). A reduced signal in labyrinthine fluids can be observed during the course of certain forms of fibrosis or in ossifications of the labyrinth. Spontaneous CPA hypersignals can be seen in teratomas and lipomas of the pontocerebellar angle, in tumors with a hemorrhagic or cystic component, and when certain foreign bodies are present (lipiodol bubbles).

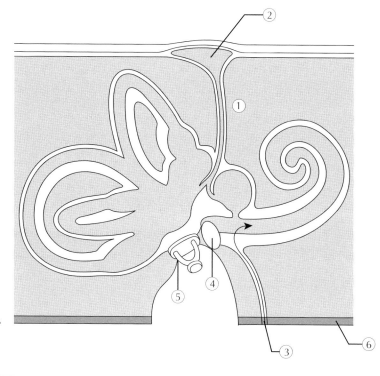

A

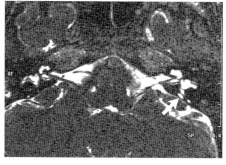

B

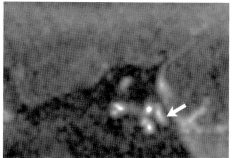

C

FIGURE 8.5 Diagram of the sensory and nonsensory parts of the inner ear.
1 : Endolymphatic canal. 2 : Endolymphatic sac.
3 : Cochlear duct. 4 : Cochlear window (round).
5 : Vestibular window (oval). 6 : Subarachnoid spaces.
7 : Dura mater. **(B)** Axial section. Slight dilatation of the left endolymphatic canal, parallel to the posterior semicircular canal (→). Hypoplasia of the modiolus. **(C)** Sagittal reconstruction: route taken by the canal and opening into the subarachnoid spaces (→). **(D)** CT scan. The vestibular aqueduct is clearly visible (→).

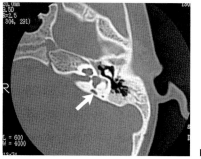

D

TABLE 8.1 Signal Anomalies in Labyrinthine Fluids and the CPA During T1-Weighted Sequences

Spontaneous Hypersignal	Reduction in Signal
Hemorrhages	Labyrinthine ossification
Lipomas	Fibrosis
Teratomas	
Calcifications	
Foreign bodies (lipiodol)	

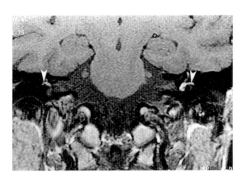

FIGURE 8.6 Spontaneous bilateral labyrinthine hemorrhage. T1-weighted MR image sequences without gadolinium. Abnormal hypersignal in the two posterior labyrinths: vestibule and anterior and lateral semicircular canals (➤).

T1-Weighted Sequence With Gadolinium Injection. A T1-weighted MRI sequence with gadolinium injection is intended to document enhancement in the acoustic–facial bundle, the labyrinth, the meninges covering the endocranial surface of the petrosal bone, or the endolymphatic sac and/or duct. Enhancement in these structures is always pathologic (Fig. 8.7).

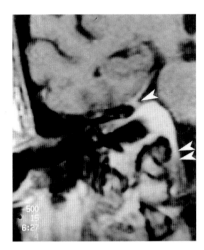

FIGURE 8.7 Coronal T1-weighted MR image sequence after gadolinium injection. Abnormal enhancement of the internal acoustic meatus due to a plaque-shaped meningioma descending into the epidural space (➤➤) and toward the jugular foramen and extending up to the tentorium cerebelli (➤). Absence of labyrinthine enhancement.

T2-Weighted Sequences With Submillimetric Sections, Echo Gradient. The endo- and perilymphatic fluids have a very high signal intensity, rendering the lamina spiralis ossea readily visible in the form of a linear intralabyrinthine hypointense structure (Figure 8.8). The modiolus appears as a hyposignal structure measuring approximately 0.3 mm; its absence is pathologic.

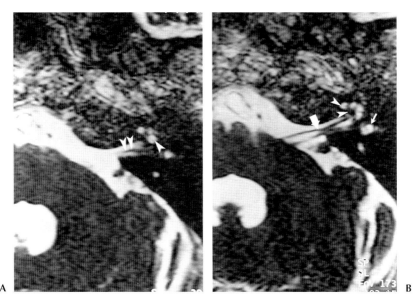

FIGURE 8.8 0.7-mm-thick axial T2-weighted MR image sections. Slices passing (A) under the facial nerve and (B) at the level of the region of the modiolus.

(A) High section; normal hypersignal from the anterior labyrinth (mesial tower); the lamina spiralis ossea is visible (➤). Behind, the ampullae of the anterior and posterior semicircular canals can be seen. In the internal acoustic meatus, the acoustic–facial packet has an intermediate signal; the utricular nerve is seen in back (➤➤). (B) Low axial section through the plane of the modiolus, which appears to be in hyposignal (➤). At the level of the internal acoustic meatus, the cochlear nerve (→) is in front of the inferior vestibular (saccular) nerve. The ampulla of the anterior semicircular canal and vestibule (→) is seen.

Sagittal Reconstruction With Multiplane Reconstructions. With sagittal reconstruction with multiplane reconstructions (MPR), the IAM and the pathway of the endolymphatic sac and conduit are able to be studied. Oblique coronal sections show the pathway of the acoustic–facial bundle and its relationship to the vascular structures of the CPA.

Maximum Intensity Projection Reconstructions. Maximum intensity projection (MIP) reconstructions are used to study the three-dimensional morphology of the labyrinth (Fig. 8.9).

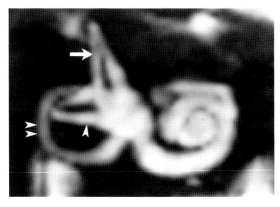

FIGURE 8.9 Cochlear–vestibular apparatus.

Maximum intensity projection reconstruction illustrating the different elements of the inner ear: the coiled cochlea, the anterior (→) and posterior (➤➤) semicircular canals, and their ampullae.

The Brainstem, the Brain, and the Cervicocranial Junction

The brainstem, the brain, and the cervicocranial junction are explored using T2 spin echo brain sequences and, for a number of these elements, using FLAIR sequences (T2-weighted with black cerebrospinal fluid), which allows good discrimination between lesions and white matter. The cervicocranial junction can also be explored using sagittal T1-weighted sequences. Sections taken after the injection of gadolinium can verify the absence of abnormal meningeal or parenchymal enhancement.

Computed Tomography Scanning

Indications for CT scanning are restricted to the study of bony labyrinthine structures to look for expanding lesions in the IAM in patients with a contraindication to MRI and for the preoperative workup of expanding lesions in the IAM (study of the temporal bone to planify surgical approach). A high-resolution CT scan without the injection of contrast material should be performed, except when there is a contraindication to MRI. The slices should be thin (0.5 to 1.5 mm) and contiguous or even sometimes overlapping to study the bony outline of the labyrinth with the minimum partial volume and the maximum clarity. High-resolution spiral CT scan using slices ≤0.6 mm actually offers good-quality multiple-plane reconstructions.

DISORDERS
Membranous Labyrinth
Congenital Anomalies

Developmental anomalies of the labyrinth can be isolated or associated with a syndrome with a number of other malformations. These anomalies can be studied by using CT scanning and T2-weighted MRI sequences with thin slices. MRI can document certain malformations that cannot be seen with the CT scan: eg, hypoplasia or aplasia in a nerve branch of the acoustic–facial packet, discontinuity in the lamina spiralis ossea. To identify a malformation in the inner ear, the different elements that make up the ear must be systematically studied, particularly:

- The vestibular and cochlear windows.
- The anterior labyrinth: Number of spirals, the development of the cochlear arrow, the visibility of the lamina spiralis ossea, the size of the cochlear conduit (normally greater than 3 mm) (using MRI) (Fig. 8.8).
- The posterior labyrinth: appearance of the vestibule ("distended" appearance that is pathologic); appearance of the semicircular canals (SCC), one or both of which can be absent, short, dilated or stenotic; appearance of the surface between the vestibule and the jambs of the lateral and anterior SCC (reduced in vestibular dysplasias); study of the development of the petrosal apex opposite the semicircular canals (dehiscence of the SCC in the subarachnoid spaces).
- The vestibular and cochlear aqueducts: The diagnosis of dilatation of the vestibular aqueduct is based on its increased size (diameter greater than 1.5 mm at mid aqueduct or greater than the diameter of the posterior SCC when used as a reference).[1] MRI studies the size and the signal of the endolymphatic sac which, when dilated, can bulge into the subarachnoid spaces accompanied by a signal change during T1- and T2-weighted sequences (Fig. 8.10).[2]

1. This disease is also called "large vestibular aqueduct syndrome" or "large endolymphatic sac anomaly."

2. MR can detect more precisely associated cochlear dysphasias.

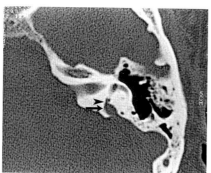
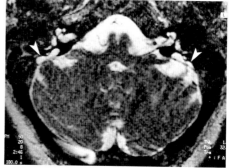

FIGURE 8.10 Significant bilateral large vestibular aqueduct syndrome.
(A) CT scan, high axial section. **(B)** Axial T2-weighted MR image. Dilatation of the aqueduct, from its origin (➤) in the vestibule up to the CPA (→). MRI demonstrates the importance of the endolymphatic sac dilatation (➤) in its extradural compartment.

- A developmental anomaly of the IAM: A diameter reduced to less than 3 mm suggests aplasia or hypoplasia of the cochlear nerve. MRI can visualize the cochlear nerve (T2-weighted sagittal oblique section) and help in determining its size in comparison to the facial nerve. When associated with an anomaly in the modiolus, a geyser ear should be suspected, especially when the size of the cochlear canal and the labyrinthine portion of the facial canal are increased.
- Abnormal orientation of the petrosal bone with sagittalization of the IAM.
- An absence of a falciform crest.

The main malformations of the inner ear are as follows:

- **Dilatations of the aqueduct of the vestibule** with a risk of geyser ear when they are associated with a disorder in the membranous labyrinth: segmental dilatation of the posterior labyrinth, insufficiently coiled cochlea, a unique cochlear cavity, or abnormal modiolus (Fig.8.11).

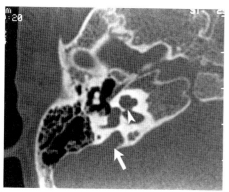

FIGURE 8.11 Large vestibular aqueduct syndrome–associated cochlear anomalies.
Significant dilatation of the aqueduct of the vestibule (→), hypoplasia of the cochlea, with wide modiolus (➤). This ear carries a risk of becoming a geyser ear.

- **Dysplasias or aplasias of the posterior labyrinth.** Dysplasia of the lateral SCC is the most frequently seen disorder and is sometimes diagnosed late. Dysplasia of the lateral SCC can produce a clinical picture of otospongiosis. The diagnosis is confirmed by the demonstration of a short, wide SCC associated with a wide vestibule. Agenesis of the SCC is seen in the CHARGE association (**Coloboma, Heart disease, choanal AtResia, Genital hypoplasia, Ear abnormalities)** and in Waardenburg syndrome (deafness, heterochromia of the iris, lock of white hair on the forehead).

- **Disorders of the anterior labyrinth,** from aplasia (Michel syndrome) (Fig. 8.12) to the presence of a unique cochlear cavity with hypoplasia of the lamina spiralis ossea (Figs. 8.13 to 8.15). Mondini syndrome consists of an incomplete cochlea containing only one and a half spirals, without a lamina spiralis ossea, forming a common tympanovestibular ramp. The detection of high-pitched auditory frequencies can be partially intact owing to the presence of the basal tower. There is no risk of meningitis because the cerebrospinal fluid of the IAM is separated from the cochlear canal.

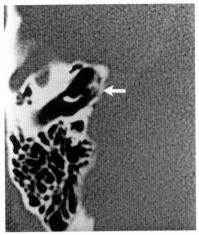
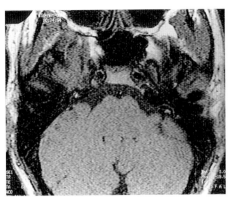

A   B

FIGURE 8.12 Michel aplasia.
(**A**) Computed axial tomography scan, axial section. (**B**) T1-weighted MR image. Aplasia of the labyrinth and the apex of the petrosal bone (→).

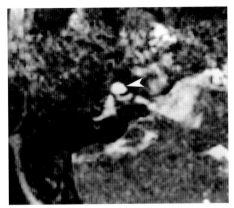
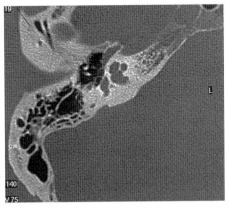

FIGURE 8.13 Congenital cochlear malformation.
MR image. Single cochlear cavity (→), hypoplasia of the lamina spiralis ossea, and wide modiolus.

FIGURE 8.14 Abnormal cochlear segmentation found during the workup for progressive deafness in an adult.
Reduced cochlear size. Partial aplasia of the osseous lamina spiralis ossea, wide modiolus. Flattened promontory.

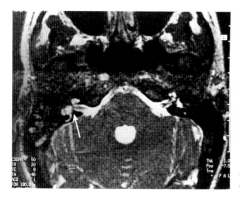

FIGURE 8.15 Posttraumatic perilymphatic fistula
(barotrauma due to a violent sound).
Congenital dilatation (→) of the vestibule was discovered.

- **Geyser ear** results from an excessive pressure into the membranous labyrinth with the presence of cerebrospinal fluid in the inner ear. Geyser ear can be associated with genetic perception deafness linked to the X chromosome. The diagnosis is based on an increase in the size of the cochlear canal associated with dilatation in the labyrinthine portion of the canal of the facial nerve and in the superior vestibular nerve. These malformations carry a risk of meningitis and of spontaneous fistula, which can appear after barotrauma or surgical exposure of the windows (Fig. 8.15).
- **Thinning of the temporal bone covering the anterior SCC**. This bony dehiscence results in deafness due to the transmission of pressure variations of CSF into the internal ear.

Labyrinthine Hemorrhages

A number of different causes, including coagulation disorders, can produce labyrinthine hemorrhage (Table 8.2). Although not visible with CT scan, the hematoma can be seen with MRI during the subacute phase in the form of a spontaneous T1 hypersignal (Fig. 8.6). Thus, MRI can play an important medicolegal role during the course of trauma to the inner ear with destruction of the labyrinth in the absence of a visible fracture on the CT scan.

TABLE 8.2 Causes of Labyrinthine Hemorrhages

Traumatic
With or without fracture
Iatrogenic
Postoperative: surgery of the window of the vestibule (oval), neurinoma surgery
Systemic Disorders
Anticoagulant therapy
Coagulation disorders
Leukemia
Small-vessel arterial disease
Intralabyrinthine fissuring tumors
Diffusion from a subarachnoid hemorrhage

Labyrinthitis

Labyrinthitis can have a number of causes: infection (viral, bacterial, syphilis) or auto-immune. Bacterial labyrinthitis can be the result of the following:

- **Eardrum disorders:** Unilateral, secondary to diffusion from a middle ear infection through the windows of the cochlea or the vestibule (Fig. 8.16).
- **Meningeal disorders:** Secondary to meningeal disease and spreading to the inner ear by the aqueduct of the cochlea or the IAM.

With MRI, the diagnosis is based on enhancement of the labyrinth during T1-weighted sequences after gadolinium injection (Fig. 8.16) and occasionally with a hypersignal from the labyrinthine fluid during T1-weighted sequences (Fig. 8.17). The disappearance of a fluid signal during T2 indicates the presence of granulomatous tissue. This tissue often calcifies.

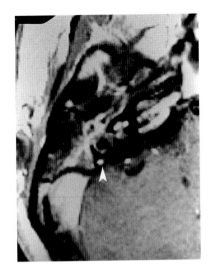

FIGURE 8.16 Labyrinthitis caused by a disorder of the eardrum. Enhancement of the anterior labyrinth and, to a lesser degree, of the posterior labyrinth. Enhancement of the endolymphatic sac (➤).

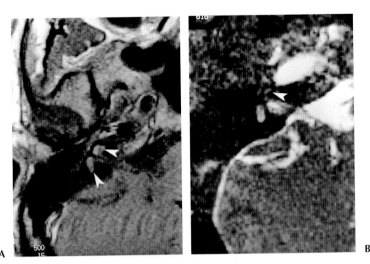

A   B

FIGURE 8.17 Calcifying bacterial labyrinthitis with fibrotic scarring.
(A) T1-weighted MR image (MRI) sequence. **(B)** T2-weighted MRI sequence. Slight, spontaneous hypersignal from the membranous labyrinth (➤) **(A)** with complete disappearance of the fluid signal intensity from the cochlea (➤) and semicircular canals during T2-weighted sequences (→, B).

The bacterial and autoimmune types of labyrinthitis produce severe, irreversible perception deafness. When bilateral, a cochlear implant can be justified (Fig. 8.17). The granuloma scar can produce stenotic calcifications in the cochlear canal that, in cases of meningitis, predominate in the basal turn, the area where the cochlear canal joins the aqueduct of the cochlea. Hyperostosis of the round window (fenestra cochlea) is frequently associated.

Endolymphatic Hydrops (Ménière Disease)

Ménière disease is generally thought to be due to an increase in the pressure of endolymphatic fluid. Imaging is used to exclude other disorders that can simulate Ménière disease. According to a number of authors, the inability to see the endolymphatic sac and conduit with MRI using thin sections during T2-weighted sequences and the finding of a reduction in the thickness of the bone between the posterior SCC and the medial wall of the petrosal bone suggest that this syndrome has a congenital origin.

Tumors of the Labyrinth

Tumors of the labyrinth are, for the most part, constituted by labyrinthine schwannomas. These tumors produce an intralabyrinthine mass-effect syndrome with a hyposignal during T2-weighted MRI sequences, an intermediate signal during T1-weighted MRI sequences, and enhancement after gadolinium injection. These tumors spread toward the two windows according to location: toward the window of the vestibule (oval) if originating in the vestibular ramp and toward the window of the cochlea (round) if originating in the tympanic ramp.

The presenting symptom of labyrinthine tumors can be the appearance of mixed deafness; they can produce a mass-effect syndrome in the middle ear when they are located close to the windows. Consequently, an isolated mass near the window of the vestibule or the cochlea should be explored with MRI (Fig. 8.18).

Bony Labyrinth

Fractures of the Labyrinth

CT scan is useful for studying the pathways of fracture lines. MRI is useful in studying blood in the labyrinth, with labyrinthine fluid showing a high signal during T1-weighted sequences. Translabyrinthine fractures are caused by a violent impact, producing a shock wave that begins at the occipital bone or the squama and spreads toward the petrosal mass.

Fractures of the labyrinth are very disabling and their main complications include:

- **Peripheral facial paralysis** caused by a hematoma compressing the geniculate ganglion or dish-pan fracture at the facial nerve.
- **A perilymphatic fistula** secondary to a fracture of the windows or disinsertion of the annulus. When the fracture line passes through the windows of the labyrinth, the fracture allows communication between the middle ear's air space and the fluids in the inner ear and can produce a perilymphatic fistula. The presence of air in the labyrinth (pneumolabyrinth) confirms the communication between the middle and inner ears (Fig. 8.19).
- **Fluid otorrhea** (sometimes rhinorrhea) that indicates a meningeal breach with leakage of cerebrospinal fluid.
- **Purulent meningitis** due to a meningeal breach. MRI may show signs of cerebrospinal fluid fistula: a linear image with a high signal during T2-weighted MRI sequences located along the fracture line, allowing communication between the middle ear and the labyrinth.

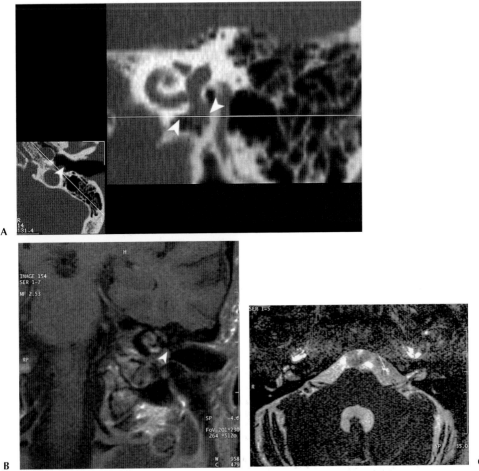

FIGURE 8.18 **Schwannoma of the cochlea protruding through the round window. MR evaluation of a sudden episode of deafness.**
(**A**) CT scan, reconstruction in the axis of the petrosal bone. (**B**) T1-weighted MR sequence after gadolinium injection. (**C**) T2-weighted MR sequence. Rounded mass (arrowhead) in the mesotympanum widening the round window (**A**), with enhancement after gadolinium injection (**B**). Enhancement of the cochlea, which loses its signal during T2-weighted MR sequences (**C**).

- **Perception deafness and vertigo** due to labyrinthine commotion or perilymphatic fistula.

Otospongiosis of the Cochlea and the Stapes Footplate

Certain forms of otospongiosis can be found during evaluation of sensoring neural hearing loss, tinnitus, or vertigo. The diagnosis can be made with CT scan, which demonstrates perilabyrinthine demineralization that sometimes extends to the posterior labyrinth and the IAM. With MRI, these forms sometimes produce a pericochlear hyposignal during T1-weighted MR sequence enhancing after gadolinium injection.

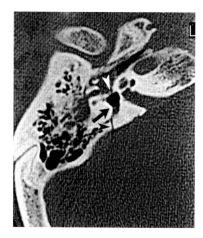

FIGURE 8.19 Fracture of the labyrinth.
Axial CT scan. Intravestibular air (→). Fracture of the footplate of the
stapes (➤).

Bone Dysplasias

Bone dysplasias are constituted by Lobstein disease, fibrous dysplasia, and Paget disease, which
can involve the otic capsule and produce sensory impairment (Fig. 8.20).

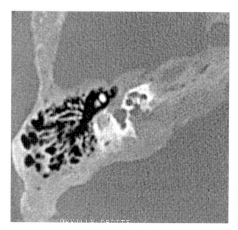

FIGURE 8.20 Paget disease.
Severe deafness and tinnitus. Perilabyrinthine demineralization
involving the entire petrosal bone but sparing the endosteal bone.

Internal Acoustic Meatus

The most frequent expanding lesions of the IAM are vestibular schwannomas misnamed "neurinomas of the acoustic nerve" (8 to 10% of all intracranial tumors, 90% of all tumors of the CPA). These
lesions consist of an intra- or extracanalar mass that has acute joining angles with the temporal
bone and a major axis that is parallel to the acoustic–facial bundle. The association of bilateral
schwannomas or a schwannoma associated with a meningioma constitute one of the criteria for
type 2 neurofibromatosis (Fig. 8.21).

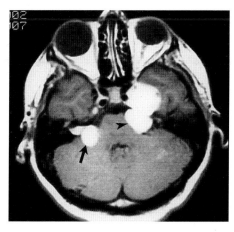

FIGURE 8.21 Multiple schwannomas, neurofibromatosis type 2.
T1-weighted MR image sequence after injection with gadolinium. Enhancement of the expanding mass in the right internal acoustic meatus (→), with the pathway of the left V nerve in its cisternal portion (➤) invading the cavernous sinus and the trigeminal ganglion.

MRI should assess tumor size or at least tumor volume (follow-up); identify the nerve from which the tumor has developed; assess its extension with respect to the porus, the anterior and posterior labyrinths, and the CPA; and finally, look for the presence of anomalies in venous development (Fig. 8.22). Evaluation of the size of the tumor is one of the most striking key points because these tumors frequently are not operated on. Therefore, measurements should be done in a reproducible manner; using the same sequence, enhanced T1-weighted sequence is the best in the case of tumor extension within the IAM. Thin sections during T2-weighted sequences should be used to look for the persistence of fluid between the tumor and the far end of the IAM to direct the surgical approach (Fig. 8.23). When no more liquid is present, the translabyrinthine approach should be used because audition can no longer be spared and the cochlear canal requires verification.

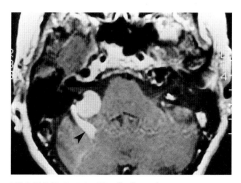

FIGURE 8.22 Vestibular schwannoma associated with an anomaly of venous development.
MR imaging. Axial section. T1-weighted sequence after gadolinium injection. Extracanalar mass growing from the posterior portion of the internal acoustic meatus, in the cerebellopontine angle, associated with a linear, tubular image (➤) and extending to the interior of the cerebellar lobe.

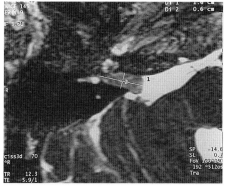

FIGURE 8.23 Intracanalar schwannoma.
MR imaging. T2-weighted, gradient echo CISS, 0.7-mm-thick axial slices. Intermediate signal mass extending to the far end of the internal acoustic meatus without any signal anomaly in the labyrinthine fluids. Extension to the modiolus imposes a translabyrinthine approach.

An expanding mass in the IAM surrounding the acoustic–facial bundle requires that the following disorders be excluded:

- **Meningioma.**
- **Hemangioma or arteriovenous malformation.** Elements in favor of these two diagnoses include: perineural diffusion surrounding the vessel–nerve element, a perpendicular extension to the nerve axis, a presence of hypersignal areas during T1 sequence, and an intraosseous extension (Fig. 8.24).
- **Lipoma fat suppression of the IAM**. T1 sequences with and without the suppression of fat signals can help in this diagnosis (Fig. 8.25).

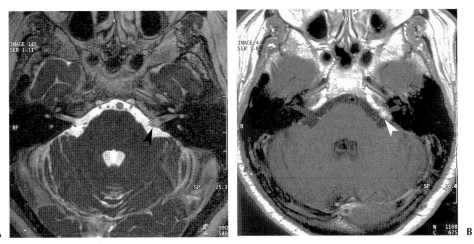

FIGURE 8.24 Hemangioma.
(A) T2-weighted constructive interference in steady state sequence. (B) T1 MR image sequence after gadolinium injection. Intracanalar mass (➤) with intraosseous spread (➤), perpendicular to the nerve axis, with enhancement after gadolinium.

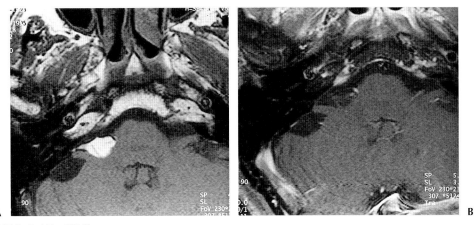

FIGURE 8.25 CPA lipoma.
T1-weighted MR image sequences without (A) and with (B) gadolinium and fat suppressed. Mass with a hypersignal during T1 (A), which is relatively homogenous, disappearing during T1-weighted sequences with fat suppressed, without enhancement after the injection of gadolinium (B).

- **Neuritis**. Nerve sheath enhancement can mimic a tumor but high-resolution T2 sequences with thin slices show that the nerve axis has a normal morphology.
- **Inflammatory meningeal disorders (sarcoidosis, intracranial hypotension, etc.), tumors (meningioma, lymphoma, metastasis)** (Fig. 8.26). The thickened meninges meet on the midline surrounding the nerve packet. Clinical presentation, multifocal meningeal enhancement, and nipplelike contours of the mass suggest the diagnosis of metastatic pachymeningitis. The lesions can spread into the labyrinth preferentially to the cochlea.

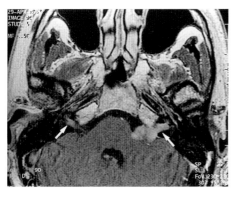

FIGURE 8.26 Leptomeningeal metastasis.
MR image. Enhanced T1-weighted sequence. Bilateral enhancement (→) of the internal acoustic meatus, extending to the cochlea. The nipplelike contour of the mass and the visibility of the right cochlear and vestibular nerves suggest the diagnosis of metastatic pachymeningitis.

Postoperative Follow-Up

After removal of a vestibular schwannoma, a baseline reference image should be performed at 3 months. A spontaneous hypersignal in the labyrinth corresponds to postoperative hemorrhage. Residual tissue in the IAM that enhances after gadolinium injection and persists during sequences with fat suppressed suggests postoperative fibrosis or residual tissue (Fig. 8.23). Enhancement due to postoperative fibrosis is transitory, disappearing during the subsequent follow-up studies, which should be yearly at first, then performed less frequently.

Residual intracanalar contrast uptake is a bad sign when tumors are nodular or when they appear secondarily or increase during subsequent follow-up studies (Table 8.3) (Fig. 8.27).

TABLE 8.3 Postoperative MR image Appearance of a Vestibular Schwannoma According to the Different Weighted Sequences Used

	T1	T1 + Fat Suppressed	T1 + Gadolinium + Fat Suppressed	T2
Fat filling	+	−	−	Intermediate
Blood	+	+	−	Intermediate
Inflammation	−	−	+	+
Residual neurinoma	Intermediate	Intermediate	+ +	Intermediate size → during follow-up

+, hypersignal; −, hyposignal.

Simple follow-up, notably in untreated patients, requires a precise assessment of the volume of the mass to be sure that the schwannoma (or meningioma) is not growing. When multiple-beam radiotherapy is used imaging is performed to determine whether there are any complications (radiation-induced lesions to adjacent nervous structures) and to monitor tumor regression. A delay of 2 years is necessary to appreciate the effect of the multiple-beam radiotherapy.

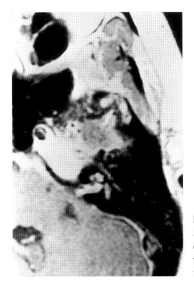

FIGURE 8.27   Follow-up for a surgically treated neurinoma.
MR image. T1-weighted sequences after the injection of gadolinium. Persistent enhancement of the internal acoustic meatus (→) extending to the labyrinth with reactionary pachymeningitis. Postoperative inflammation regressed during the subsequent follow-up examination.

Cerebellopontine Angle

Lesions of the IAM extend from or originate near the CPA. During the course of mass lesions in the CPA, imaging can assess the effect of the mass on the brainstem, the persistence of a liquid interface between the mass and the brainstem, any rotation in the brainstem, displacement of midline structures, and compression of the IVth ventricle (obstructive hydrocephalus).

To determine the origin of a tissue lesion in the CPA, the following disorders must be considered:

- **Schwannoma** (Fig. 8.28): Elements in favor of this diagnosis include a mass with sharp contours, a cystic component, acute connecting angles, the absence of overflow in front of the facial nerve, and the absence of bone involvement. The axis on which a schwannoma develops is related to the nerve origin of this tumor; a schwannoma of the acoustic–vestibular bundle goes toward the IAM, whereas a schwannoma of the VII nerve travels toward the geniculate ganglion.

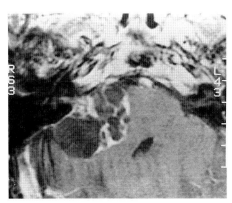

FIGURE 8.28   Cystic vestibular schwannoma with intra- and extracanalar development.
T1-weighted MR image sequence with gadolinium injection. Expanding mass overflowing the anterior plane of the internal acoustic meatus (IAM) with acute connecting angles with the meninges and the cerebellopontine angle. Homogeneous enhancement with cystic components. The intracanalar extension spreads to the far end of the IAM. Deformation of the IVth ventricle with compression of the lateral recessus. Rotation of the brainstem.

- **Meningioma,** which spreads in front of the facial nerve, contains gentle sloping connecting angles and thickening in the endocranial meninges.
- **Leptomeningeal metastasis** (Fig. 8.26) is suggested by the clinical presentation, multiple lesions in the cranial nerves, involvement of the base of the skull, a "dart-like or fringed" appearance on its borders, and a rapid clinical course.
- **Epidermoid cysts** (Fig. 8.29) are hypointense during T1 and hyperintense during T2 sequences, similar to the signal coming from cerebrospinal fluid. Gradient echo, diffusion, and FLAIR MRI sequences can be helpful for differentiating epidermoid cysts from arachnoid cysts (Fig. 8.30).

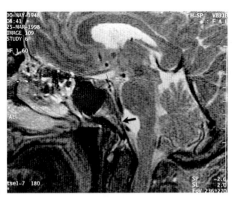
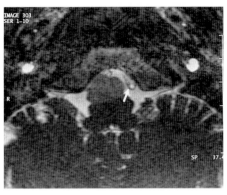

A   B

FIGURE 8.29   Epidermoid cyst.
Right paramedian mass that is hyperintense in T2 MR image (MRI), nondissociable from the signal coming from the cerebrospinal fluid (→), with an intermediate signal in echo gradient. Compression of the basilar artery (white, →). **(A)** MRI, T2-weighted spin echo sequence, sagittal section. **(B)** MRI, T2-weighted echo gradient sequence, axial section (→).

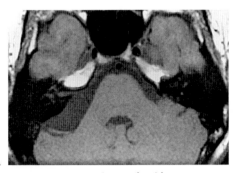
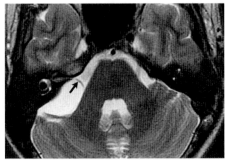

A   B

FIGURE 8.30   Compressive arachnoid cyst.
MR image. T1-weighted sequence, axial section **(A)**. T2-weighted sequence **(B)**. Hypointense mass with a signal similar to cerebrospinal fluid. During T1 **(A)**, the cyst is more intense than the cerebrospinal fluid. During T2, the cyst is only visible by the compressive effect it produces on the acoustic–facial packet (→).

- **Tumors of the endolymphatic sac** (Fig. 8.31) are seen mainly in patients with Von-Hippel-Lindau disease. These hypervascular tumors strongly take up contrast material, contain cystic components that are frequently hyperintense, and have a bivalve development in the CPA as well as along the petrosal bone via the intrapetrous vascular structures. They present with flow void.
- **Jugular glomus tumor.**

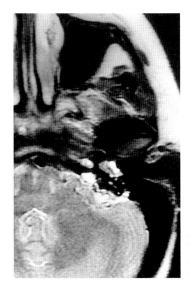

FIGURE 8.31 Tumor of the endolymphatic sac.
T2-weighted sequence. Mass exhibiting a heterogeneous, areolar hypersignal centered on the area of the endolymphatic sac, extending to the CPA, the apex of the petrosal bone, and the middle ear.

Vascular disorders of the CPA should be assessed with Doppler ultrasound, MRI, and magnetic resonance angiography (MRA). Vascular disorders of the CPA may impinge on the neurosensory axis by producing a mass-effect (aneurysm), a vascular loop (Fig. 8.32), or ischemia secondary to stenosis in one of the branches going to the labyrinth or the vestibulocochlear nuclei (Fig. 8.33). MRA (native sections) can be used to assess stenosis of the basilar trunk. Thin sections during T2-weighted echo gradient sequences can allow visualization of a contact between the vascular and nerve structures. To be considered pathologic, a vascular loop must be demonstrated in two different spatial planes and distort the vascular–nerve axis.

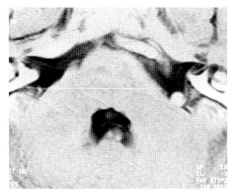

FIGURE 8.32 Vascular loop.
Megadolicho basilar artery. Vascular loop impinging on the exit point of the VIII nerve (→). Distortion of the brainstem and the lateral recessus of the bulb.

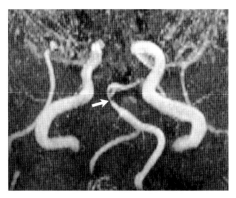

FIGURE 8.33 Ischemic lesion in the vestibulocochlear nuclei due to basilar artery stenosis (→).

Intra-axial Lesions

Intra-axial lesions are constituted by disorders involving the intra-axial pathway of the auditory tracts. Lesions in the cerebral auditory fibers result in bilateral perception deafness that predominates on the contralateral side of the axial lesion.

Imaging

The best procedures for diagnosing chemodectomas and for localizing multiple lesions are CT scan and MRI, and better yet, isotope scan using meta-iodobenzylguanidine (MIBG) marked with iodine 131 or iodine 123.

Tympanojugular chemodectomas are located near the jugular foramen and/or the tympanic cavity; carotid chemodectomas are found near the carotid bifurcation; and vagal chemodectomas are located behind the styloid process of the temporal bone, too high to be carotid chemodectomas and too low to be tympanojugular chemodectomas.

During CT scan, chemodectomas are well-limited, spontaneously hypodense tumors that massively and rapidly enhance after the injection of contrast material. When chemodectomas are located in the tympanojugular area, thin sections along the base of the skull and the petrosal allow assessment of the tympanic cavity and allow assessment of any tumor-related bone destruction.

During MRI, chemodectomas elicit a homogeneous, hypointense signal during T1 and a heterogeneous "salt and pepper" appearance during T2 sequences. Gadolinium injection is followed by massive and rapid enhancement. During the course of tympanojugular or vagal chemodectomas, MRI allows complete assessment of tumor spread.

Points to Remember

The vestibular ramp (window of the cochlea) and the tympanic ramp (window of the vestibule) communicate through the helicotrema, a channel of the lamina spiralis ossea located at the summit of the cochlea.

Because it has a terminal-type vascularization, the labyrinth is vulnerable to ischemia.

In the IAM, the facial nerve is located cephalad and in front, the cochlear nerve is caudate and in front, and the vestibular nerves are behind.

Only thin-section T2-weighted MRI sequences can effectively exclude expanding masses within the canal or the labyrinth.

The endolymphatic sac opens into the middle of the endocranial surface of the petrosal bone.

The modiolus or "columella" constitutes the central osseous axis of the cochlea, where the cochlear nerve passes. It forms the lamina spiralis ossea.

Lesions in the jugular foramen have an effect on the inner ear.

A normal CT scan, even after the injection of contrast material, does not completely exclude an expanding process within the canal.

Pachymeningitis can give an appearance resembling tumor in the IAM.

Always completely assess the two IAM: bilateral schwannomas or an associated meningioma in the IAM is strongly suggestive of type 2 neurofibromatosis.

Always include an assessment of the supratentorial region: the presence of a schwannoma or a meningioma suggests the diagnosis of type 2 neurofibromatosis in a subject more than 30 years old.

After surgery for a tumor in the IAM, contrast uptake within the canal can simply be related to postoperative fibrosis.

THE VERTIGO SYNDROME

D. Soulie

Vertigo is a **subjective symptom** of the **false sensation** of the movement of objects with respect to the subject or of the subject with respect to objects. It is defined by a **concomitant objective sign**: vestibulo-ocular nystagmus. Vertigo is due to a disorder in the vestibular system: the posterior labyrinth, vestibular nerve, and the centers dealing with the integration and treatment of signal. These disorders cause false information to be transmitted to the centers concerned with equilibrium, in contradiction to the other sources of information, which deny any real movement at all. The sensation of vertigo is due to this **sensory conflict.**

The radiologic assessment of vertigo constitutes the last stage in the list of diagnostic procedures (Figs. 8.34 and 8.35). CT scan and MRI furnish complementary information: CT scan is indicated for assessing osseous or calcified structures, whereas MRI is used for exploring liquid-filled structures and soft tissue. A functional approach to the vestibular system and proprioceptive and visual efferents will be based on future developments in functional MRI. Doppler ultrasound should not be systematically performed, except during the checkup of positional vertigos when a vascular origin is suspected.

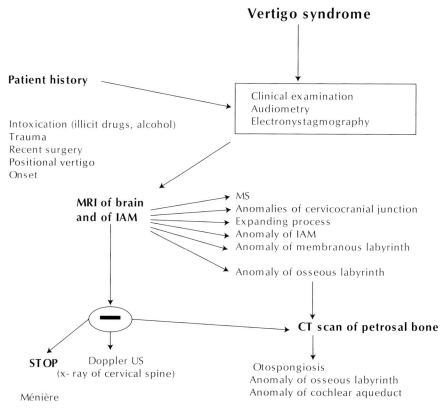

FIGURE 8.34 Assessment in a patient presenting with a vertigo syndrome.

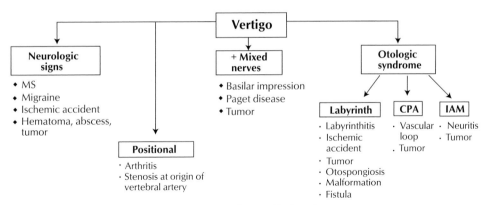

FIGURE 8.35 **Principal causes of vertigo that can be detected by imaging.**

Imaging Procedures

CT scan should be considered as a second-line procedure designed to look for a congenital petrosal anomaly, trauma, dysplasia, or dystrophia, with the exception of posttraumatic vertigo, during which CT scanning can effectively assess the fracture line and its relationship to the labyrinth.

The MRI protocol consists of the following sequences:

- A sequence exploring the entire head using 2 echoes: proton-density weighted and T2 or FLAIR.
- A high-resolution T2-weighted sequence using thin slices along the IAM and the labyrinth.
- A T1-weighted sequence, with and without the injection of contrast media, using thin slices along the IAM and the labyrinth.

Disorders

Central Vertigo

Ischemic strokes of the brainstem and the posterior fossa are most often secondary to an occlusion of the vertebral artery or the posteroinferior cerebellar artery (PICA). When an ischemic stroke occurs, vertigo is rarely isolated and is usually accompanied by a procession of neurologic signs related to the lesions in the bulb. On MRI, cerebellar infarction appears as an area with a hyperintensity T2 and hypo- or isointensity T1 with peripheral gyriform enhancement after the injection of gadolinium, covering an arterial vascular territory (Fig. 8.36). MRI results can be negative when transitory ischemia is the cause. Isolated vertigo can be the first clinical sign of ischemia and lesions in the territory of the anteroinferior cerebellar artery (the middle cerebellar peduncle and the anteroinferior portion of the cerebellar hemisphere) may only appear later with imaging. Sometimes a spontaneous or secondary (cervical manipulation, trauma) vertebral dissection is found.

In 5 to 7% of cases of **multiple sclerosis** (MS), a vertigo syndrome can constitute the inaugural symptom (Fig. 8.37).

All **expanding processes**, within or outside the cerebellum, can produce vertigo by a direct mass effect on the brainstem, the cerebellum itself, the vestibular nuclei, or the association tracts (Fig. 8.38).

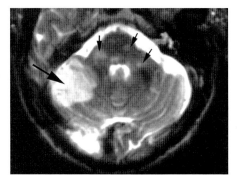

FIGURE 8.36 MR image.
T2-weighted axial section. Multiple hypersignals (→) of variable size during T2 in the right cerebellar hemisphere and the brainstem: multifocal ischemic cerebrovascular accidents in a patient who had thrombosis in the right carotid and vertebral arteries.

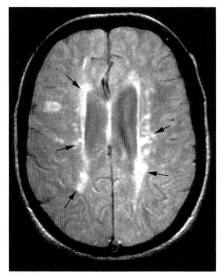

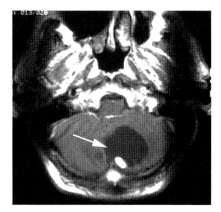

FIGURE 8.38 MR image.
Axial T1 section after gadolinium injection. Tumor mass in the cerebellum that is essentially cystic (→), containing nodular tissue on its wall that enhances after the injection of contrast material: hemangioblastoma.

FIGURE 8.37 MR image, axial section.
Periventricular hypersignals that are typical of multiple sclerosis.

Anomalies of the Cervicocranial Junction

Vertigo can be associated with lesions in the last cranial nerves, cervical pain, and headache that is often precipitated by maneuvers that increase the pressure in the cerebrospinal fluid.

The diagnosis is based on the finding of basilar impression (standard profile film, MRI). MRI can directly show an anomaly in the position of the tonsilla cerebelli and, occasionally, a syringomyelia (Fig. 8.39).

The Cerebellopontine Angle (CPA)

An arterial, vascular loop can compress the vestibulocochlear nerve at its origin. The relationships between the nerve and blood vessels can studied by using thin sections during three-dimensional T2 sequences with multiple reconstructions and magnetic resonance angiography. A megadolichobasi-

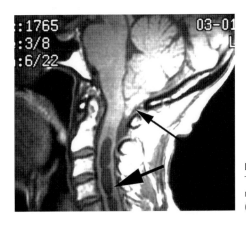

FIGURE 8.39 Sagittal section MR image.
T1 sequence. Herniation of the tonsilla cerebelli into the foramen
magnum (→) due to a malformation in the cervico-occipital junction
(Chiari I), underlying syringomyelia.

lar artery can sometimes cause vertigo: MRI can identify the abnormal vessel, dilated or tortuous,
and describe its pathway in relation to the nerves.

Expanding processes in the CPA include the following:

- **Schwannomas of the VIII nerve** are the most frequent tumors of the CPA in adults (60%
  of these tumors). Most often, they develop from the Schwann cells in the inferior
  vestibular nerve.

- **Schwannomas that develop in other nerves in the CPA** (V and VII nerves) can also
  compress the vestibulocochlear nerve.

- During MRI, **meningiomas** show a wide meningeal base of implantation with intense
  enhancement after the injection of gadolinium, the presence of calcifications (25% of
  the cases), and associated osseous anomalies (which are easier to see on a CT scan).

- MRI appearance of **primitive cholesteatomas** is characteristic with a polygonal or irregular
  contour. These tumors have a tendency to infiltrate. Their signal is heterogeneous and
  slightly hyperintense during T1 relative to the cerebrospinal fluid, producing a marbled
  appearance. The signal of cholesteatomas is similar to cerebrospinal fluid during T2.
  During FLAIR, these tumors present a well-individualized hypersignal in the hyposignal of
  the cerebrospinal fluid. There is no enhancement after the injection of contrast media. The
  diffusion coefficient is increased (diffusion MRI).

- **Dermoid cysts** are heterogeneous and rare.

- **Metastases and leptomeningeal carcinosis** are suggested when a primary tumor is
  found and when multiple localizations exist. MRI is the most sensitive procedure for
  identifying parenchymatous or meningeal, diffuse or localized contrast uptake.

Internal Acoustic Meatus

Any disorder of the IAM can first appear with a vertigo syndrome:

- Schwannoma
- Nerve inflammation (viral neuritis, sarcoidsis) (Fig. 8.40)
- Hemangioma or meningioma

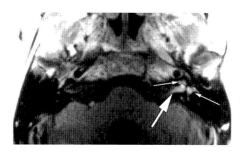

FIGURE 8.40 Neuritis.
T1 sequence after gadolinium injection, axial section. Enhancement of the vestibulocochlear nerve in the left internal acoustic meatus (→), associated with enhancement in the intralabyrinthine fluids of the cochlea and the vestibule (→); this aspect suggests neuritis (immunodepressed patient) and association with labyrinthitis.

The Labyrinth and Its Environment

The Membranous Labyrinth

Tumors of the membranous labyrinth (Fig. 8.41), the endolymphatic sac, and bacterial, viral, or autoimmune labyrinthitis can cause vertigo. All of these elements produce enhancement in the signal of the labyrinth or the endolymphatic sac during T1 sequences after the injection of gadolinium (Fig. 8.40).

Nearby Tumors

Lesions in the semicircular canals or in the vestibule cause vertigo. Diverse tumors can invade the membranous labyrinth: cholesteatomas of the middle ear, cholesterol granuloma of the petrosal bone, or a tumor in the IAM (Fig. 8.41).

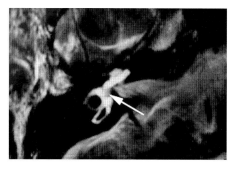

FIGURE 8.41 MR image.
T2 sequence, axial section. Nodular image with a hyposignal in the vestibule (→) corresponding to an intralabyrinthine schwannoma.

Osseous Labyrinth

Otospongiosis (Fig. 8.42), fibrous dysplasia, Lobstein disease, and Paget disease can cause a vertigo syndrome with tinnitus and deafness. CT scan is the first-line procedure for studying these disorders; MRI can assess their effects on the membranous labyrinth.

Congenital Malformations

Malformations are frequently encountered and often remain undiagnosed until adulthood. The most commonly seen malformation is dilatation of the endolymphatic sac or wide labyrinthine aqueduct syndrome (Fig. 8.43), which is associated with progressive perception deafness, vertigo, and loss of equilibrium. The diagnosis can be made by using imaging that shows dilatation of the sac and of the endolymphatic duct, most often bilateral, isolated, or associated with another anomaly of the membranous labyrinth. More rarely, these procedures show dilatation or hypoplasia of a semicircular canal or dilatation of the vestibule related to Mondini dysplasia. Exceptionally, a perilymphatic fistula is diagnosed in an infant presenting with fluctuating deafness, a vestibular

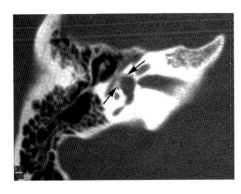

FIGURE 8.42 Computed axial tomography scan, axial section.
Hypodensities in the perivestibular area and opposite the fistula ante fenestram (→); foci of otospongiosis.

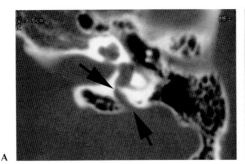

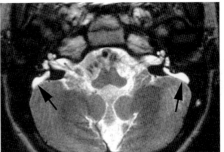

A   B

FIGURE 8.43 Congenital malformations of the labyrinth.
CT scan, axial section (**A**). MR image, T2-weighted sequence, axial section (**B**). Dilatation of the sac and the endolymphatic duct (→) with a fluid hypersignal during T2. The sac is much more dilated than it appears in the CT scan.

syndrome, and occasionally, recurrent meningitis. Dilatation of the aqueduct of the cochlea is characteristic but remains exceptional.

Trauma to the Petrosal Bone

Trauma to the petrosal bone or the windows of the membranous labyrinth (posttraumatic or postoperative depression in the middle ear) can cause vertigo that usually resolves rapidly in a few weeks.

MRI can show evidence from intralabyrinthine hemorrhage in rare cases of labyrinthine commotion without fracture. Posttraumatic perilymphatic fistulas are diagnosed clinically; findings on imaging are inconstant. Perilymphatic fistula can be suggested during CT scan by a fracture line passing through the windows associated with a more or less important filling of the middle ear (Figs. 8.44 and 8.45) that sometimes involves only a recessus and that is variable over time. Intralabyrinthine air during the acute phase is a characteristic finding.

Middle Ear

During the course of middle ear disorders, the clinical examination immediately suggests the cause of the vertigo syndrome; CT scan is only indicated for the pretherapeutic checkup.

A **cholesteatoma** of the middle ear can be accompanied by a lesion in the inner ear when there is lysis in the osseous labyrinth. A cholesteatoma can even produce a veritable fistula. This complication is frequent and is found in 10% of all cholesteatomas. Most often, the lateral semicircular canal is involved.

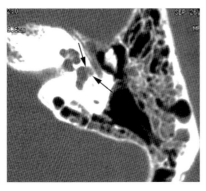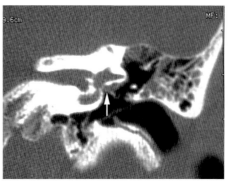

FIGURE 8.44 Petrosal trauma.
CT scan, axial (**A**) and frontal (**B**) sections. Petrosal trauma. Soft tissue density in the mastoid cells without a visible fracture. Soft tissue density (→) filling the area of the oval window of the vestibule, corresponding to an accumulation of fluid from the fracture of platinum.

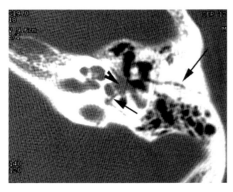

FIGURE 8.45 CT scan, axial section.
Transverse fracture of the petrosal radiating to the vestibule with a multilobed opacity filling the area of the window of the vestibule (➤), changing when moving to the frontal position, and corresponding to a fluid accumulation from a fracture of the processus palatinus maxillae; the fracture line is on the promontory (→).

When a complication after surgery on the **platinum** for otospongiosis is suspected, a CT scan should be performed.

An **aberrant carotid artery** or a **pro-eminent jugular gulf** can be the cause of transmission deafness, with or without tinnitus and a pseudovertigo syndrome. The diagnosis can be made with a CT scan of the petrosal bone.

Vertigo Caused by Disorders of the Cervical Spine

The cervical spine origin for vertigo is not universally accepted, with the exception of vertigo secondary to trauma involving the upper cervical vertebra or when a malformation in the craniocervical junction is present. Most often, the checkup for positional vertigo related to neck rotation or extension, associated with hearing impairment and posterior "helmet" headache, remains negative. Plain radiographs and CT scanning can exclude cervical osteophytosis of the foramen and constitutional anomalies (cervical rib, megatransversal process, muscular hypertrophy)that can impinge on the vascular axis.

In summary, CT scan and MRI, can be used to explore the labyrinth and the vestibular pathways. The numerous causes of vertigo and the lack of specificity in the clinical findings indicate that a complete assessment of the head and the cervico-occipital junction should be performed. Even though imaging fails to make the diagnosis in nearly two of three patients, this is improving because of better cooperation between clinicians and radiologists. In addition, radiologists are learning more about the different causes that need to be looked for and the most appropriate techniques to use to diagnosis these causes. Clinicians must clearly identify all of the possible diagnoses to exclude to be able to order the most appropriate imaging procedure:

- **MRI should be considered a first-line procedure** in both peripheral and central vertigo. CT scan is indicated only as a complement to MRI, to assess osseous structures or search for calcified tissue.

- **MRI should be used as a complement to CT scan** when the patient has a history of inner ear surgery.

- **CT scan should be considered a first-line procedure** when there is chronic inflammation of the middle ear, a history of recent or old trauma, or middle ear surgery; MRI is useful in assessing extension to the inner ear and for determining the cause.

- **CT scan should be ordered when MRI is impossible:** For example, when the patient is claustrophobic, presents an absolute contraindication, or when extreme urgency exists. In this case, the CT scan should be performed with the injection of contrast material and should include the same target zones as those already described for MRI.

TINNITUS

J. Thiebot, F. Callonnec, and L. Brunereau

Tinnitus is a very frequent disorder. It consists of the perception of a sensation of sound localized in one or both ears, or even inside the skull, when no external sound vibration has entered the auditory apparatus. The psychological effects of tinnitus are often dramatic, partly owing to the sleeping difficulties they engender.

Two main types of tinnitus should be distinguished:

- **Subjective:** By far the most frequent type, sounds are only perceived by the patient and often the cause and mechanism remain unknown. In 50% of the cases, tinnitus is bilateral and most often the sounds are high-pitched and not very intense; hearing deficit is often associated.
- **Objective:** Less frequent sounds are audible by the examiner. These sounds are the consequence of a vibratory phenomenon located in the craniocervical region, within or outside the ear.

Tinnitus is termed "pulsating" when sounds are synchronous with cardiac rhythm: they can also be either subjective or objective.

Etiologies

Subjective tinnitus can be due to lesions situated at any level of the auditory pathways: the external ear (Fig. 8.46), the middle ear, the inner ear (Fig. 8.47), the IAM, the CPA, and the central nervous system (Table. 8.4). Considering the numerous different possible causes, the choice of which procedure, sometimes invasive, is conditioned by the severity of the disability occasioned by the tinnitus. This is especially important because in 50% of cases, no anomaly is discovered. In addition, treating the cause is not always curative; tinnitus can persist even after the destruction of the inner ear.

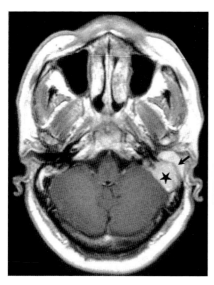

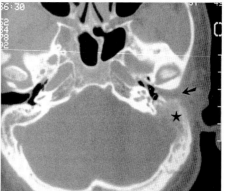

A

B

FIGURE 8.46 Plasmocytoma in the left external ear. MR image (**A**) and CT scan (**B**) during T1-weighted, axial sections after injection of contrast material. Bone lysis in the mastoid (★) and the posterior wall of the external acoustic meatus (EAM). Tissue filling in the EAM, clearly visible.

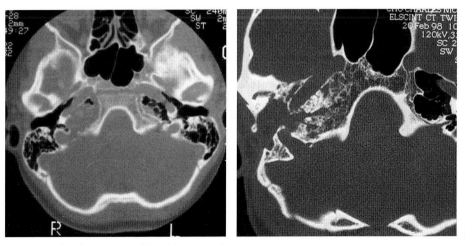

A   B

FIGURE 8.47 Chondrosarcoma of the right petrosal apex.
Clinical presentation: 10-year-old patient with right facial paralysis and nonpulsating subjective tinnitus. Normal auditory caval on examination. Computed tomography scan, axial sections **(A, B)**. Ballooning lesion in the right petrosal apex with partial lysis of cortical bone. Disappearance of the pneumatization of the apical cells. Extension to the right petrosphenoid synchondrosis.

TABLE 8.4 Etiologies of Subjective Tinnitus

Regional
Dental or sinus infection
Nasal obstruction
Disorder of temporomandibular joint
Internal Acoustic Meatus
Neurinoma of VIII
Neuritis: Varicella herpes zoster
Central Nervous System
Subjective postconcussion syndrome
External Ear
Cerumen plug
External otitis
Osteoma
Middle Ear
Otospongiosis
Serous otitis
Chronic otitis
Cholesteatoma
Inner Ear
Ischemic syndromes
Ménière's disease
Traumas: blast, barometric, presbyacousia
Toxic: Hg, barbiturates, CO, Pb, cisplatine.
Labyrinthitis: infectious, cholesteatomas, sudden or fluctuating deafness.

Add all causes of pulsatile tinnitus.
No etiology is found in approximately 50% of cases.

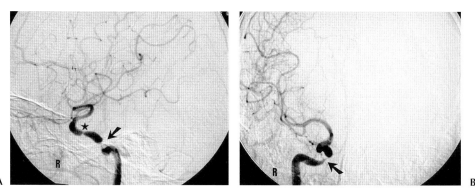

FIGURE 8.48 Stenosis of the left internal carotid artery within the petrosal.
Clinical presentation: 70-year-old diabetic patient with hypertension who reported sudden right-headed whistling. Arteriography in lateral **(A)** and frontal views **(B)** show severe, double stenosis in the left internal carotid artery within the petrosal (→) and the carotid siphon (★).

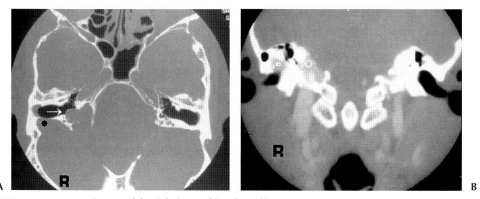

FIGURE 8.49 Pro-eminence of the right internal jugular gulf.
Clinical presentation: right pulsatile, disabling tinnitus with a bluish appearance in the posterior wall of the right external acoustic meatus. **(A)** Computed axial tomography (CT) scan, axial section at the external acoustic meatus. High-riding right jugular bulb. Bulging in the middle ear (→). Bone dehiscence (★) of the posterior wall of the conduit and the tympanic cavity. **(B)** CT scan, coronal section after the injection of iodine passing through the jugular bulbs, showing widening of the gulf of the sinus and the right jugular vein and its impact on the adjacent bone.

Objective tinnitus, in contrast, is more specific. It is very often pulsatile; when it is not pulsating, it can be muscular in origin (in the form of a clicking noise) and is generally due to clonus in the ossicular muscles.

A definite cause is more often discovered in objective tinnitus. Two thirds of cases are caused by the following:

- Tympanojugular glomus tumors
- Benign intracranial hypertension
- Carotid atherosclerosis (Fig. 8.48)

Pulsatile tinnitus can vary with breathing (tubal gaping) or with cardiac rhythm, suggesting a vascular anomaly in the region (Table 8.5). Changes in the flow within an artery or a vein (Fig. 8.49) secondary to stenosis, compression, arterial hypertension, or an arteriovenous **shunt** (Fig. 8.50) can also cause tinnitus (Fig. 8.51).

TABLE 8.5 Vascular Etiologies of Pulsatile Tinnitus

Arterial causes
  Congenital
    Aberrant internal carotid artery
    Persistent stapedial artery
  Acquired
    Atherosclerotic stenosis, turbulent flow
    Fibromuscular dysplasia
    Dissection of the internal carotid artery
    Aneurysm in the intrapetrous portion of the internal carotid artery
    Increased cardiac output (anemia, thyrotoxicosis, pregnancy)

Venous causes
  Congenital
    Diverticulum of the jugular bulb
    Dehiscence of the jugular bulb
  Acquired
    Stenosis of the transversal and sigmoid sinus
    Benign intracranial hypertension
    Condyloid or emissary vein

Arteriovenous causes
  Vascular
    Dural fistula
    Intracranial fistula
  Tumor
    Glomus tympanicum
    Jugulotympanic glomus
    Glomus jugular
    Meningioma
    Paget disease

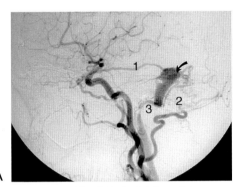

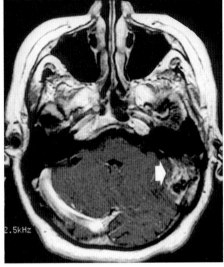

FIGURE 8.50 Dural fistula in the left lateral sinus.
Clinical presentation: 45-year-old patient who had objective,
pulsating tinnitus with left hemicrania. A history of severe
head trauma 10 years ago. **(A)** Left carotid angiogram; lateral
view. Fistula in the left lateral sinus (↗) irrigated by meningeal
branches of the middle meningeal artery (1) and the occipital
artery (2). Ipsilateral venous drainage with severe stenosis of
the jugular bulb (3). **(B)** MR image. T1-weighted axial section
after injection of contrast material: asymmetry of the lateral
venous sinuses (left hypersignal related to increased flow).

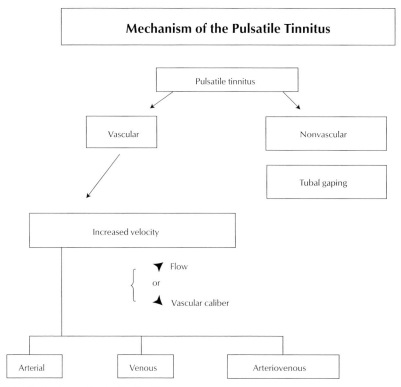

FIGURE 8.51 Mechanisms of pulsatile tinnitus.

Pathophysiologic Hypotheses

To explain tinnitus, a number of hypotheses have been advanced: eg, disorders of neuromediators, imbalance in ion exchanges in the cochlea, cellular tetany. Nevertheless, Corti organ, particularly sensitive to anoxia and ischemia, is probably a very frequent component in many cases of tinnitus.

Clinical Management (Fig. 8.52)

Patient History

Benign intracranial hypertension should be suspected when a young, obese, female patient reports tinnitus, headache, and/or visual disturbances. The association of high blood pressure, history of ischemic episodes, and cardiovascular risk factors should suggest carotid atherosclerosis. When tinnitus appears after severe head trauma, intracranial dural fistula must be excluded. Dissection of ICA should be suspected when the patient reports headache, tinnitus, neck pain, and/or ischemia.

Clinical Examination

The otoscopic examination is used to look for an anomaly of the tympanic membrane, particularly a bluish eardrum, which suggests a vascular lesion. However, this finding can also be encountered in serous otitis or cholesterol granulomas (Table 8.6).

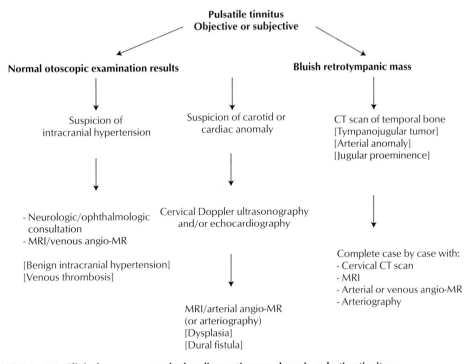

Pulsatile tinnitus
Objective or subjective

Normal otoscopic examination results

Bluish retrotympanic mass

Suspicion of
intracranial hypertension

Suspicion of carotid or
cardiac anomaly

CT scan of temporal bone
[Tympanojugular tumor]
[Arterial anomaly]
[Jugular proeminence]

- Neurologic/ophthalmologic
consultation
- MRI/venous angio-MR

[Benign intracranial hypertension]
[Venous thrombosis]

Cervical Doppler ultrasonography
and/or echocardiography

Complete case by case with:
- Cervical CT scan
- MRI
- Arterial or venous angio-MR
- Arteriography

MRI/arterial angio-MR
(or arteriography)
[Dysplasia]
[Dural fistula]

FIGURE 8.52 Clinical assessment and other diagnostic procedures in pulsating tinnitus.

TABLE 8.6 Differential Diagnosis of a Bluish Tympanic Membrane

Arterial causes	Infectious–Inflammatory causes
Aberrant internal carotid artery	Cholesterol granuloma
Lateralized internal carotid artery	Serous otitis
Intrapetrous arterial aneurysm	**Tumors**
Venous causes	Tympanic or tympanojugular glomus
Dehiscence of the jugular bulb	

Audiometry and Auditory Evoked Potentials (AEP)
Radiologic Procedures

- Radiologic procedures should include CT, MRI, MRA, Doppler ultrasound, and arteriography.

Procedure Techniques

Computed Tomography Scan

CT is especially useful in assessing bony and vascular structures, according to clinical findings and other diagnostic results:

- Millimetric or submillimetric slices in a bone window of temporal bone in axial or coronal direct acquisition or helicoid sections, with ultrahigh definition.

- And/or angio CT scan after a bolus injection. Spiral acquisition should be performed with 3-mm slices or smaller, reconstructed every 1.5 mm in a parenchymatous window, with a distance of 1 mm or smaller between slices.

When a bluish mass is discovered during otoscopic examination, the carotid canal (location, wall), the pneumatization of the mastoid cells and the cavity, and the jugular foramen should be assessed with CT scan. CT has a preponderant role considering the difficulty in excluding the differential diagnoses and the risk involved when these bluish lesions are biopsied.

MR Image/Magnetic Resonance Angiography Protocol

MRI should be performed using thin slices (3 to 4 mm), in axial and coronal planes with the injection of contrast material to study all the anatomic areas from the torcular to C5. T1-weighted spin echo sequences should be used preferentially. MRA is performed during time of flight or during phase contrast. Some operators use rapid sequences with the injection of contrast material. In all cases, the partitions should be studied during the arterial and/or venous phases, according to the presaturations. The native slices must be meticulously studied and the field of view necessarily wide so that a fistula is not overlooked. MRI and MRA are essentially used to study cervical internal carotid and petrosal arteries, lateral sinuses, and jugular veins.

Cervical Color Doppler Ultrasound

Cervical color Doppler ultrasound is only helpful when its results are positive. It is effective for the diagnosis of extracranial fistulas.

Arteriography

Arteriography should not be systematically performed. It can be indicated in the preoperative assessment of glomus tumors or carotid stenosis, with or without embolization. If the diagnostic procedures remain negative and the tinnitus is disabling and objective, carotid and vertebral arteriography can be performed in order to exclude fibromuscular dysplasia or an arteriovenous fistula.

A Few Unusual Causes: Tinnitus Due to Vascular Lesions

This type of tinnitus classically has either a systolic and/or diastolic pulsation. Patients report a "blowing sound in the ear" synchronous with cardiac rhythm. The murmur can be subjective or objective. When it is objective, a vascular disorder in close contact to the skull and the dura mater should be suspected (arteriovenous shunt).

The principal causes that should be excluded are:

- Cervical and cerebral arterial dissections
- Intracranial dural fistulas
- Chemodectomas

Cervical and Cerebral Arterial Dissections

Generalities. Cervical and cerebral dissections are the cause of approximately 1% of all cerebral ischemias. They occur spontaneously or occur after trauma to the cervical spine (strangulation, manipulations, highway accidents). Underlying vascular disease, fibromuscular dysplasia, Marfan syndrome, or Ehlers-Danlos syndrome are risk factors for dissection; in addition, vascular loops are also frequently found.

Two types of dissection are classically distinguished:

- **Subintimal**, which is responsible for stenotic (60%) or occlusive (20%) dissections
- **Subadventitial**, which is responsible for aneurysmal forms

Clinical Manifestations. Dissections can cause two types of signs at onset, which are present to varying degrees in the majority of cases:

- **Local signs:** headache, neck pain, Horner syndrome, dysphagia, and of course, pulsatile tinnitus
- **Ischemic signs** are present in 84% of cases; cerebrovascular accidents or transient ischemic accidents and are secondary to embolism or hemodynamic causes.

Imaging. The diagnosis of cervical and cerebral dissections is based on a triad: neurovascular ultrasound, MRI with MRA, and finally, conventional angiography. MRI coupled with MRA should include T1- and T2-weighted axial sequences covering the entire lengths of the internal carotid and vertebral arteries, an MRI of the brain using a T2-weighted axial sequence or even a T1-weighted sequence after injection of gadolinium, and one or a number of MRA sequences. Only sequences using the time-of-flight technique have been validated in the literature; with a sensitivity of 95% and a specificity of 99%. The imaging findings in carotid dissection include widening in the external diameter of the artery, reduction in the internal lumen, and occasionally, direct visualization of the hematoma in the form of a suspended hypersignal. To be able to see the hypersignal, the hematoma must be in the "methemoglobin" stage, meaning that the dissection is already 4 to 5 days old. One of the causes of false-negative findings during time-of-flight MRA is carotid dissection in its very early stage. Other causes of misdiagnosis are the presence of a short dissection (<1 cm) or the concomitant existence of a complex vascular loop. It is likely that, in the future, MRA with the injection of contrast material will supplant the time-of-flight technique for assessing cervical arterial dissections.

Intracranial Dural Fistulas

Generalities. Dural fistulas are arteriovenous shunts located in the dura mater of the skull or the spine. Within the skull, dural fistulas are supplied by meningeal branches of the external and internal carotid arteries and/or of the vertebral arteries. They drain into one or a number of dural sinuses and/or into one or many cortical veins. They are most often located in the lateral sinus.

The cause of dural fistulas remains unknown: in 30% of the cases, patient history reveals trauma, upper respiratory infection complicated by empyema, or even cerebral thrombophlebitis; however, in the remaining cases (70%), the patient's medical history in unremarkable.

Clinical Presentation. The age of onset is around 50 years. The first signs include minor signs (headache, pulsating tinnitus, ophthalmologic signs) and major signs (epileptic seizures, a focal neurologic deficit, hemorrhage, intracranial hypertension). Some types of dural fistulas carry a risk of hemorrhage.

A classification that correlates to the clinical prognosis has been suggested: type I fistulas have a spontaneously benign clinical course without the appearance of any major clinical signs and can forego treatment. In contrast, fistula types 2 to 5 are associated with major clinical signs and imperatively require treatment (embolization, surgery). The principal prognostic factor for cerebromeningeal hemorrhage is involvement of cortical vein.

Imaging. Imaging techniques like Doppler ultrasound, MRI coupled with MRA, and CT scan can supply only indirect evidence for diagnosing dural fistulas: the presence of a dilated venous network located in the dural wall of the sinus that opacifies early and allows communication between the venous network and the neighboring arterial network (internal or external carotid). These peripheral signs can be seen on MRA or CT scan native sections. Conventional cerebral angiography should be performed in every case to confirm the diagnosis and to determine the type of fistula. Angiography should include selective catheterization of the external and internal carotid and vertebral arteries and can be concluded by a therapeutic procedure.

Chemodectomas

Generalities. Paraganglions are cells originating in the neural crest that are distributed throughout the entire body and play a hemodynamic role in utero through the intermediary of catecholamine secretions. After birth, the majority of these paraganglion cells spontaneously regress,persisting only in the adrenal glands (adrenal medulla) and the vessels of the neck and heart (baroreceptors).

All tumors that develop from paraganglions are termed "paragangliomas." They are mostly benign tumors and are malignant in only 3 to 20% of cases. Below the arch of the aorta, paragangliomas are pheochromocytomas; above the aortic arch, they are chemodectomas.

Chemodectomas are hypervascular tumors that normally do not secrete catecholamines. The three most frequent localizations are as follows:

- **Tympanojugular chemodectoma** (48%). Tympanojugular chemodectomas predominate in women and can occur at any age. They make up two thirds of all petrosal tumors. They are found in the jugular foramen or in the tympanic cavity along Jacobson nerve, the tympanic plexus, or Cruveilhier Arnold nerve and are rarely bilateral. Clinically, they are accompanied by pulsatile tinnitus, hearing deficit, vertigo, and sometimes an auricular discharge. When viewed through an otoscope, the intratympanic part of the tumor gives a bluish appearance to the eardrum (Table 8.6).

- **Carotid chemodectoma** (35%). Carotid chemodectomas are found along the carotid bifurcation, where they push back the internal and external carotid arteries. They are bilateral in 5% of cases. The presenting sign can be a palpable neck mass, dyshagia, or cough.

- **Vagal chemodectoma** (11%). Vagal chemodectomas are often associated with other forms of chemodectoma (carotid, tympanojugular) and are located beneath the base of the skull along the pathway of the vagus nerve. The clinical onset can be paralysis of the X, IX, or XI nerves or a lesion in the cervical sympathetic nerves.

9

Normal Appearance and Disorders of the Mixed Nerves: IX, X, and XI

M. Gayet-Delacroix, F. Benoudiba, and F. Domengie

The IX, X, and XI nerves have similar proximal origins and pathways, beginning in the brain stem and traveling to the nasopharyngeal vascular space after traveling through the jugular foramen. Beyond the nasopharynx, their routes diverge. Impairment in these nerves is often associated with other disorders in the neighboring areas.

CLINICAL ASPECTS

Disorders of the IX are rarely isolated; they produce otalgia and impaired speech and swallowing. The vomit reflex is eliminated.

The clinical signs associated with **disorders of the XI** are often late appearing and include lowering of the shoulder and atrophy of the sternocleidomastoid or trapezius muscles. These findings are frequently seen during the clinical examination but are rarely present at onset.

Disorders of the X are the most frequently occurring owing to the length of this nerve. Dysphonia is the principal symptom. When the clinical examination of the larynx reveals a tumor, imaging and a complete patient physical examination can help to determine the stage as a function of the extension. When the examination reveals impairment in one or both vocal cords, a meticulous clinical assessment can help to orient imaging procedures according to whether the lesion is **proximal** or **distal**: proximal if the lesion involves the X nerve between the brain stem and the hyoid bone, distal if it is between the hyoid bone and the aortopulmonary window on the left and the subclavian artery on the right. These anatomic and functional criteria are important because they help guide imaging.

Proximal lesions are accompanied by dysphonia, lung aspiration, dysphagia, and clinically, by deviation of the uvula toward the unaffected side and elimination of the vomit reflex. When both laryngeal and oropharyngeal symptoms are present, the clinician should search for lesions in the other cranial nerves, from the IX to the XII nerves.

Distal lesions are related to an isolated lesion in the X and/or the recurrent nerves and produce dysphonia and lung inhalation due to laryngeal dysfunction; however, there are no oropharyngeal symptoms or any association with other clinical signs suggesting a disorder in other cranial nerves.

Proximal lesions of the IX, X, and/or XI nerves are located in the brain stem, the posterior basal cistern, the skull base, the jugular foramen, and/or the suprahyoid vascular space.

Distal lesions of the X nerve are found in the subhyoid vascular space, the mediastinum, the left aortopulmonary window, and the two tracheoesophageal subhyoid angles (lesion in the recurrent nerve) if only lesions in the neck and brain are considered.

IMAGING

Imaging should be performed as a function of the clinical findings: MR image (MRI) is the best procedure for studying a proximal lesion in the X nerve, regardless of whether it is associated with a disorder in the IX or XI nerves. MRI has better sensitivity than computed axial tomographic (CT) scanning for studying the brainstem, the cistern of the skull base, and the nasopharynx. T2-weighted axial sequences and high-resolution T2 sequences with and without gadolinium injection should be performed and eventually completed with fat suppressed in the axial and/or frontal planes (Fig. 9.1). CT scanning can be a useful complement for a precise assessment of the skull base using a high-resolution bone filter, direct axial and frontal acquisition, or reformatting after axial volume acquisition. Also, a new ultrasonic technique for studying nerves along the extracranial pathways using high-frequency (12–15 mHz) sounds has been developed. With this technique, the most peripheral nerves, like the X nerve, can be followed all along their respective pathways (Fig. 9.2).

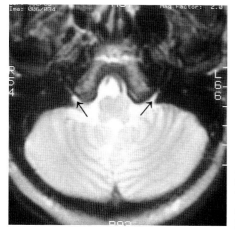

FIGURE 9.1   Normal anatomy. MRI T2 section: mixed nerves in the foramen jugular.
T2 section passing through the posterior fossa clearly showing the arachnoid sheathing (→) around the IX, X, and XI nerves during passage through the nerve cleft of the jugular foramen.

A distal lesion in the X nerve is best studied with CT scanning from the base of the skull to the aortopulmonary window using volume acquisition and the automatic injection of iodine contrast material. Reformatting is possible.

CT scanning can also precisely assess the brainstem, the pathways of the nerves in the basal cistern, the jugular foramen, the supra- and subhyoid vascular space, the tracheoesophageal space, and the left mediastinum up to the aortopulmonary window. CT scanning can also be used to assess additional lesions secondary to the motor nerve lesion. The presence of muscular atrophy and fatty degeneration of muscle tissue that is easily explored in the sternocleidomastoid or the trapezius muscles and that is more difficult to demonstrate objectively in the constrictor muscles of the pharynx or the laryngeal muscles suggests an old nerve lesion.

Some images in the larynx can be secondary to lesions in the X nerve; these include displacement of the vocal cords to a paramedian position, a dilated ventricle, bending of the arytenoepiglottic fold, dilatation in the piriform sinus, and reduced density or size of the laryngeal muscles. These findings should be interpreted with caution; they are very helpful when a number of them are seen together, whereas one of these findings seen alone can be encountered in normal conditions (see Fig. 9.5).

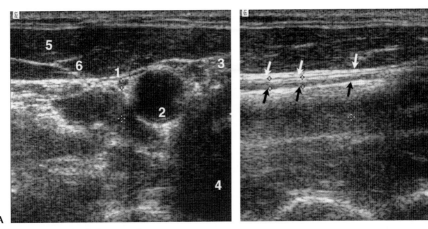

FIGURE 9.2 Cervical ultrasound.
(**A**) Axial ultrasound section using a 10-mHz probe showing the close relationship between the vagus nerve (1) and the internal carotid artery (2). (**B**) Sagittal ultrasound section (with the same probe). The vagus nerve is hypoechogenic, has a bundled appearance, and is surrounded by a hyperechogenic envelope (→). (3) The right loboisthmian junction, (4) the trachea, (5) the muscle plane, and (6) the internal jugular vein are also seen.

DISORDERS

The principal disorders will be grouped together according to their locations.

In the Brainstem

The most frequently encountered disorders in the brain stem are caused by vascular (ischemia or hemorrhage), demyelinating, and/or inflammatory lesions or tumors (primary or secondary metastasis). A lesion in a cranial nerve can go unnoticed when part of a life-threatening clinical picture.

In the Basal Cistern

The most frequent lesions in the basal cistern are inflammatory and infectious (Fig. 9.4). MRI demonstrates leptomeningeal enhancement long the nerve sheaths. This appearance is the same regardless of the cause or of the infectious agent involved. Leptomeningeal metastasis also has this same appearance.

Besides metastases, lymphomas, schwannomas, meningiomas, and epidermoid cysts may also be seen (Fig. 9.3). Vascular causes are more rare and include a megadolichovertebral artery and aneurysm in the vertebral or posteroinferior cerebellar artery. Angio MR image often can be used to determine the diagnosis, thus avoiding the use of conventional arteriography.

In the Jugular Foramen, the Base of the Skull, and the Suprahyoid Vascular Space

Tumor disorders predominate in these areas, whether they are malignant (spread from a cancer of the cavum, lymphoma, chondrosarcoma, or petrosal tumor) or benign (paraganglioma, schwannoma, or meningioma) (Figs. 9.6 to 9.10).

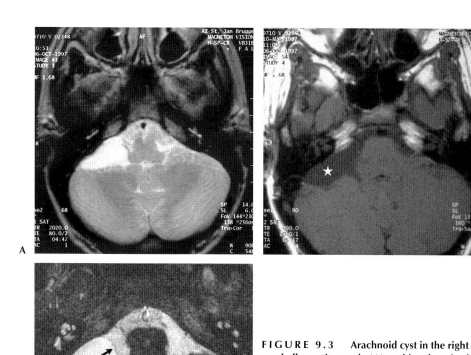

FIGURE 9.3 **Arachnoid cyst in the right cerebellopontine angle (★) pushing the mixed nerves (→).**
(A) T2 axial turbo spin echo section. **(B)** T1 axial spin echo section. **(C)** Axial constructive interference in steady state section.

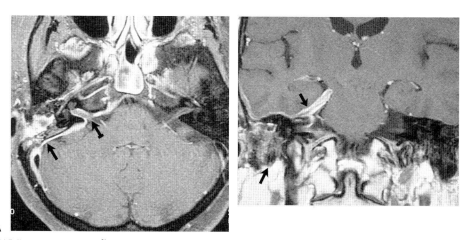

FIGURE 9.4 Wegener disease.
Progressive facial paralysis with secondary involvement of the right IX and X nerves in a 56-year-old patient. Meningeal contrast uptake at the base of the skull (→) with uptake in the right jugular foramen (→) and near the facial acoustic packet. The diagnosis of Wegener's disease was confirmed by biopsy. **(A)** Axial SE T1 section following gadolinium injection. **(B)** Coronal SE T1 section following gadolinium injection.

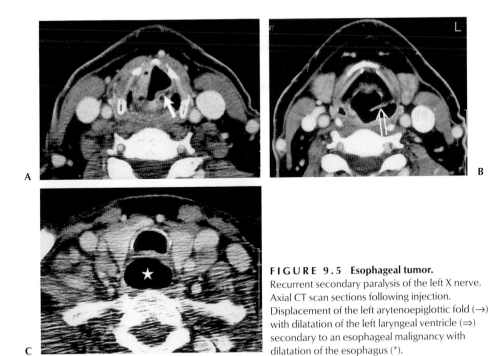

FIGURE 9.5   Esophageal tumor.
Recurrent secondary paralysis of the left X nerve.
Axial CT scan sections following injection.
Displacement of the left arytenoepiglottic fold (→)
with dilatation of the left laryngeal ventricle (⇒)
secondary to an esophageal malignancy with
dilatation of the esophagus (*).

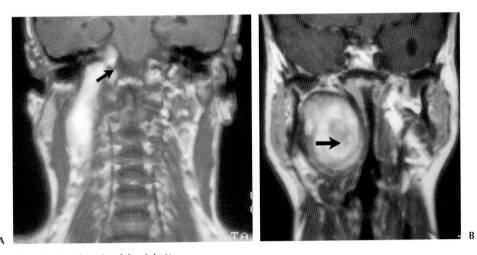

FIGURE 9.6   Neurinomia of the right X nerve.
Coronal T1 sections with gadolinium. Tumor process in the vascular space extending to the right jugular foramen (→) with
homogeneous uptake of contrast material, pushing the pharyngeal wall.

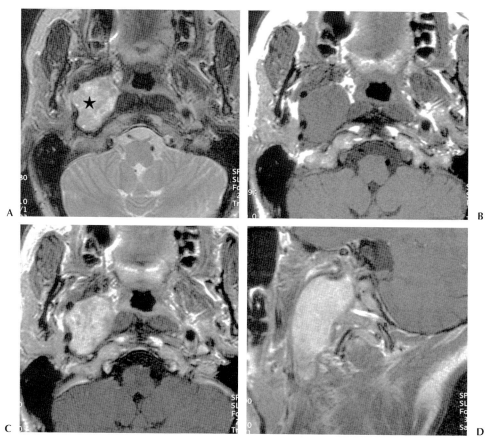

FIGURE 9.7   Paraganglioma of the X.
Paralysis of the IX, X, XI, XII, and sympathetic nerves in a 52-year-old patient. Tissue process located in the right retrostyloid space (*) extending from the jugular foramen to the C2–C3 level and developing between the jugular and carotid veins during T1 hyposignal, T2 hypersignal with well-limited contrast uptake, suggesting a paraganglioma of the X nerve. **(A)** Axial T2 section. **(B)** Axial T1 section. **(C)** Axial T1 section with gadolinium. **(D)** Sagittal T1 section with gadolinium.

MRI is more effective than CT in assessing malignant tumors, especially for studying spinal cord invasion and soft-tissue spread, particularly to the infrapetrous area, which is always difficult to see during CT scanning. Paragangliomas have a typical appearance (Figs. 9.7 to 9.10); they show very intense enhancement after gadolinium injection. When they are large enough, they contain central hypointensities ("**flow voids**") related to the presence of vascular elements. Bone invasion to the jugular foramen is frequent. CT scanning can be helpful in demonstrating the characteristic appearance of destruction at the level of the jugulocarotid wall. When looking for multiple paragangliomas (Fig. 9.10), especially in their familial form, the entire cervical regions should be studied.

The most frequently seen type of schwannoma occurs in the X (Fig. 9.6). When the Schwannoma travels through the jugular foramen, the osseous limits always remain very regular, in contrast to what is seen in paragangliomas. Meningiomas are more rare and the bone involved at the base has the same appearance as that seen in paragangliomas.

Infectious causes are mostly due to necrotic otitis externa when it extends beyond the external acoustic meatus, producing osteomyelitis of the base of the skull that can spread to the parapharyngeal spaces. MRI and CT scanning are often complementary modalities in these indications.

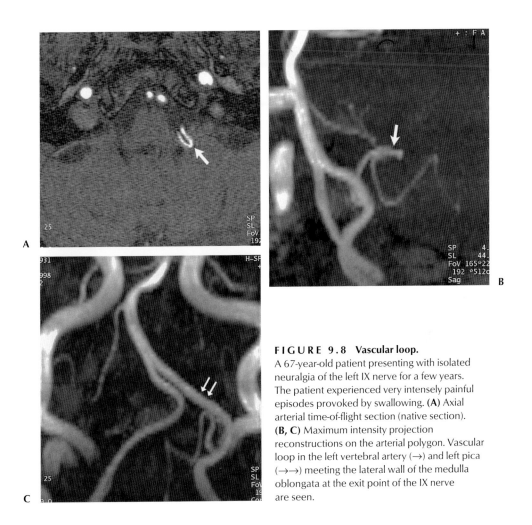

FIGURE 9.8 Vascular loop.
A 67-year-old patient presenting with isolated neuralgia of the left IX nerve for a few years. The patient experienced very intensely painful episodes provoked by swallowing. **(A)** Axial arterial time-of-flight section (native section). **(B, C)** Maximum intensity projection reconstructions on the arterial polygon. Vascular loop in the left vertebral artery (→) and left pica (→→) meeting the lateral wall of the medulla oblongata at the exit point of the IX nerve are seen.

Vascular etiologies are much less frequent and include dissection in the internal carotid artery, vascular loop (Fig. 9.8), and thrombosis of the jugular vein, which should not be misdiagnosed because of the pseudotumor appearance related to asymmetry in the diameter of the internal jugular veins at the foramens (Fig. 9.11) and to flow changes (Fig. 9.12).

At the Infrahyoid or Mediastinal Level

At the infrahyoid or mediastinal level, lesions to the X nerve are isolated and distal. They can be classified into thyroid and nonthyroid etiologies, but in both these situations tumors are the most frequent cause. **Thyroid lesions** are essentially constituted by malignant or benign tumors. Iatrogenic lesions to the recurrent nerve are often secondary to thyroid or parathyroid surgery. **Nonthyroid causes** of infrahyoid-level lesions are dominated by epidermoid carcinomas of the upper respiratory and digestive tracts, and either CT or MRI can be used to determine tumor spread and lymph node involvement. In the mediastinum, the principal lesion to the left X nerve is bronchopulmonary carcinoma, which directly invades the nerve or compresses it, either because of the primary tumor itself or because of associated mediastinal adenopathies. Non-Hodgkin's lymphoma

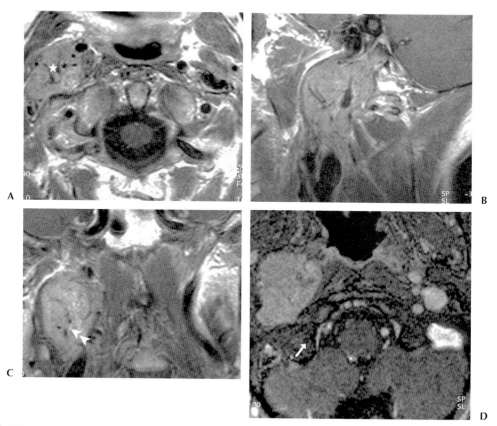

FIGURE 9.9 Paraganglioma of the X.
Patient with a modified voice with difficulty in swallowing and impaired singing for a few months. The clinical patient examination showed paralysis of the mixed nerves and of the right XII nerve. Voluminous tissue mass is centered in the carotid space (★), extending to the jugular foramen (→) and up to the carotid bifurcation. Intense enhancement with contrast material is seen with serpiginous areas in a flux hyposignal (➤➤). Enhancement was caused by a paraganglioma of the X nerve. **(A)** T1 axial section after gadolinium injection. **(B)** T1 sagittal section after gadolinium injection. **(C)** Coronal T1 section after gadolinium injection. **(D)** Axial arterial time-of-flight section.

or other secondary adenopathies can also be the cause. Vascular etiologies (aneurysm of the thoracic aorta, widening of the left pulmonary artery or the left atrium) are more rare.

A lesion in the IX nerve that produces ear pain, termed secondary, may be due to a malignant tumor in the base of the tongue or the tonsils.

Isolated impairment of the XI nerve is most often due to a nerve lesion secondary to unilateral or bilateral radical curettage.

Imaging for these three cranial nerves is closely related to the quality of the clinical assessment. Lesions in the X nerve are often the first signs of a disorder. The results of the patient examination should immediately orient the clinical search towards a high, proximal, or low distal lesion and, consequently, should be a guide for subsequent imaging.

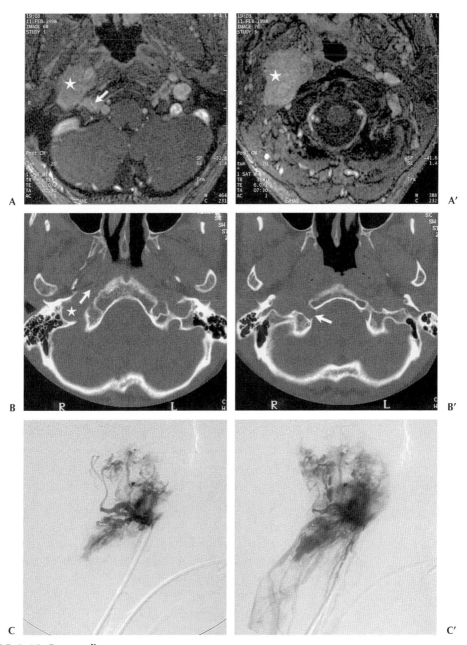

FIGURE 9.10 Paraganglioma.
Patient with no remarkable medical history presented with difficulties in singing and reported a nasal-sounding voice for 4 to 5 years. For a few months, the patient had trouble swallowing both liquids and solids. Pulsating tinnitus was confirmed by auscultation. Clinical patient examination showed paralysis of the right IX, X, and XII nerves. **(A, A')** MR image of the base of the skull: 3-mm T1 axial spin echo sections after gadolinium injection. A large, hypervascularized tumor is seen projecting into a very enlarged jugular foramen at its nerve cleft containing the IX, X, and XI nerves with a little prolongation to the hypoglossal foramen, which is enlarged (→). **(B, B')** CT scan sections of the base of the skull with a bone window. Jugular gulf (★), enlarged nerve cleft (↗), and enlarged hypoglossal foramen (→) are seen. **(C, C')** Hyperselective arteriography of the right ascending pharynx (initial arterial time and a little later) showed very significant hypervascularization. After embolization, exeresis was performed. Note that the ascending pharyngeal artery participates in the vascularization of the last four cranial nerves (IX, X, XI, and XII).

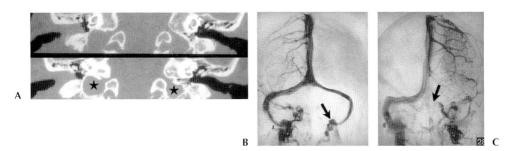

FIGURE 9.11
(**A, B**) Asymetry of the jugular vein with hypoplasia of the left jugular vein. (**C**) Thrombosis of the left jugular vein.

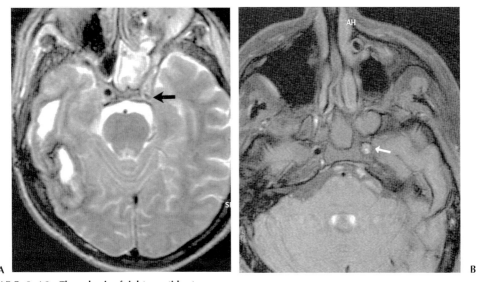

FIGURE 9.12   Thrombosis of right carotid artery.
A patient with severe head trauma with right temporal hemorrhagic contusion. Appearance of right X and XII nerve paralysis. T1 hyposignal and T2 hypersignal suggest thrombosis of the carotid artery (→); this was confirmed by arteriography, which demonstrated right carotid thrombosis with a clearly visible thrombus within the lumen (★). (**A**) T2 turbo spin echo axial sections. (**B**) T1 spin echo axial section with fat suppressed. (**C, D**) Three-dimensional reconstructed arteriography. (**E**) Arteriography.   *(continues)*

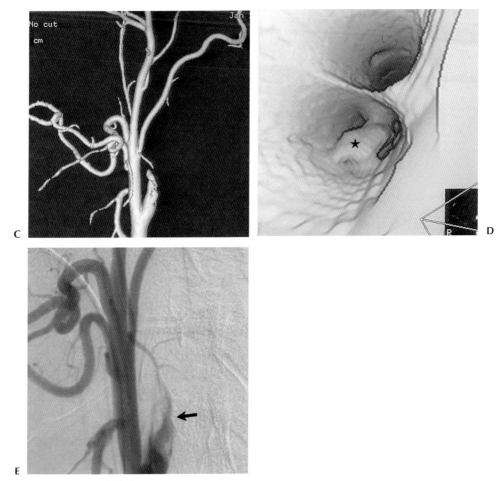

FIGURE 9.12 *(concluded)*
(C, D) Three-dimensional reconstructed arteriography. **(E)** Arteriography.

Hypoglossal Nerve (XII)

C. Iffenecker and M.-C. Petit-Lacour

EXPLORATION AND NORMAL APPEARANCE

Radiography

Standard radiography has lost much of its usefulness. However, radiography can still be helpful in assessing trauma (e.g., fracture of the condyle, atlanto-occipital dislocation).

Computed Axial Tomographic Scanning

CT scanning is especially useful in studying bone lesions because it can explore the hypoglossal canal with millimetric slices (Fig. 10.1). It can also be useful in exploring the XII nerve in the extracranial pathway and is a rough screening procedure for lesions in the intracranial portion of this nerve.

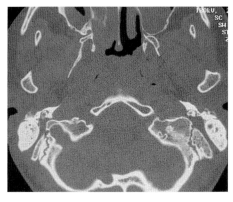

FIGURE 10.1 Hypoglossal foramen.
Computed axial tomographic scan with bone window; axial section showing the two hypoglossal foramens (→).

MR Image

MR image is the gold-standard procedure. MRI should be performed by using axial and coronal sections, as well as parasagittal sections oriented along the nerve's pathway in the hypoglossal canal. Inframillimetric T2 sections (constructive interference in steady state, three-dimensional fast spin echo) or 2- to 3-mm T2 spin echo or T1 spin echo sections should also be used. Gadolinium injection should be used when necessary.

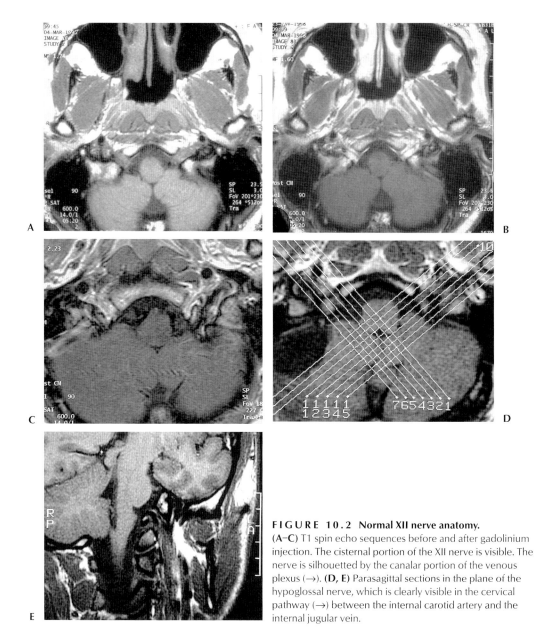

FIGURE 10.2 Normal XII nerve anatomy.
(A–C) T1 spin echo sequences before and after gadolinium injection. The cisternal portion of the XII nerve is visible. The nerve is silhouetted by the canalar portion of the venous plexus (→). (D, E) Parasagittal sections in the plane of the hypoglossal nerve, which is clearly visible in the cervical pathway (→) between the internal carotid artery and the internal jugular vein.

The procedure should study the entire pathway of the XII nerve (Fig. 10.2):

■ The supratentorial level: The supratentorial level includes the nucleus of the hypoglossal nerve that receives fibers from the inferior portion of the contralateral ascending frontal convolution (pathway of the tractus corticonuclearis = frontonuclear tractus).

■ The bulb: The bulb includes the nucleus of the XII nerve extending along almost all of its height.

■ The bulbar cistern: The bulbar cistern is where the XII nerve passes behind and lateral to the vertebral artery.

- The hypoglossal canal: The hypoglossal canal is in the occipital bone, where the XII nerve appears in silhouette during T1 after the injection of gadolinium by the venous plexus (Fig. 10.2A and B).
- The carotid space: In the carotid space (naso- and oropharynx), the XII nerve is poorly visible but a solid understanding of anatomy can help the examiner search for a lesion along the pathway. In the upper portion, this nerve is located behind the vessels, which are intimately associated with the mixed nerves. At the naso-oropharynx, the XII nerve passes between the internal carotid artery and the jugular vein, then travels in front of the carotid artery. At the mandible, the XII nerve passes under the posterior belly of the digastric muscle.
- The sublingual space: In the sublingual space, the XII nerve passes between the mylohyoid and the hypoglossal muscles.

DISORDERS

The XII nerve provides motor innervation to the tongue and unilateral paralysis produces deviation of the tongue toward the unaffected side at rest and a deviation toward the paralyzed side when the tongue is projected forward (Tables 10.1 and 10.2). Progressively, atrophy of the tongue with fatty involution appears on the affected side, which can be easily seen during T1 MRI hypersignal (Fig. 10.3). All of the intrinsic and extrinsic muscles of the tongue are affected except for the mylohyoid and the anterior belly of the digastric muscle, both of which are innervated by the V3 nerve. The XII nerve also innervates the infrahyoid muscles.

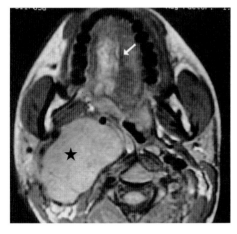

FIGURE 10.3 Neurinoma of the right XII nerve in the right retrostyloid space (★).
T1 fat hypersignal secondary to paralysis of the right XII nerve of the right-half of the tongue (→).

TABLE 10.1 Localization of the Anomaly of the XII Nerve and Clinical Symptoms

Localization	Side of Deviation	Fasciculations	Involvement of Atrophy	Laryngeal Muscles
Supranuclear	Contralateral to the lesion	No	No	No
Nuclear	Ipsilateral to the lesion	Yes	Yes	No
Infranuclear				
Above C1	Ipsilateral to the lesion	Yes	Yes	No
Below C1	Ipsilateral to the lesion	Yes	Yes	Yes

TABLE 10.2 Etiologies of Paralysis to the XII Nerve as a Function of the Localization of the Lesion

Lesion Level	Etiologies
Supranuclear	Tumors Infectious causes: abscess Inflammatory causes: multiple sclerosis Vascular causes: ischemia, hemorrhage
Brainstem	Tumors Vascular causes: hemorrhage or infarction Infectious causes: abscess, infectious mononucleosis Inflammatory causes: multiple sclerosis Other causes: acute polioencephalitis, amyotrophic lateral sclerosis
Subarachnoid pathway	Tumors: primary tumors in the nerve (neurinoma), local compression (meningioma, metastasis) Vascular causes: aneurysm of the vertebral artery, arterial ectasia, meningeal hemorrhage Infectious causes: meningitis of the skull base (tuberculosis) Craniovertebral junction: subdislocation (rheumatoid arthritis), Chiari malformation
Hypoglossal canal	Tumors: primary tumor (meningioma, chordoma), or secondary tumor from the occipital bone, jugular glomus tumor, tumor spread from the nasopharynx Bone compression: malformation of the junction, occipital fracture Infectious causes: spread from necrotic otitis externa Others: Paget disease, fibrous dysplasia
Peripheral pathway Nasopharyngeal carotid space	Tumors: tumors of the tonsils, the parotid gland, tumor extension to lymph nodes, neurinoma of the mixed nerves, paraganglioma Vascular causes: dissection of the internal carotid, aneurysm, internal jugular thrombophlebitis Infectious causes: occipito-atloid dislocation, nerve section from a penetrating neck injury Bone compression: suboccipital Pott disease, malformation of the occipito-atloid junction
Sublingual space Tongue	Tumors: carcinoma (base of the tongue, floor of the mouth) Infectious causes: infection of the sublingual space

Bilateral, total paralysis of the tongue is accompanied by impaired phonation, mastication, and deglutition. During the acute phase, muscular denervation can mimic a mass in the tongue because of edema (T1 hyposignal, T2 hypersignal, enhancement after gadolinium, and hypertrophy).

The hypoglossal nerve can be injured along the entire pathway. Patient history and physical examination indicating damage to other cranial nerves or the long pathways can be important for localizing the lesion. When the infrahyoid muscles are also involved, a lesion in the anastomotic branch of the XII nerve and C1 (C2C3) roots is suggested (Table 10.1).

Lesions in the Central Nervous System

Clinical Aspects

Supranuclear Paralysis. Lesions may be unilateral with hemiplegia. These lesions are associated with involvement in the contralateral tongue secondary to a corticosubcortical lesion (frontoparietal operculum or frontonuclear fibers). Lesions may also be bilateral, producing pseudobulbar syndrome from a lesion in the two frontonuclear tracts. *Bulbar syndrome* associates ipsilateral paralysis of the XII nerve with contralateral hemiplegia that spares the face. *Jackson syndrome* associates paralysis of the XI, X, and XII nerves with unilateral paralysis of the velum palati, the vocal cord, the sternocleidomastoid muscle, the trapezius, and paralysis of one half of the tongue.

Etiologies

Three principal etiologies of lesions in the central nervous system should be distinguished:

- Vascular causes (hemorrhage, infarction) (Fig. 10.4) in hypertensive, atherosclerotic patients
- Tumors
- Infectious causes (abscess) and inflammatory causes (multiple sclerosis)
- Lesions may also be due to other disorders such as acute polioencephalitis, syringobulbia, and amyotrophic lateral sclerosis.

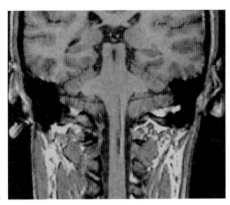 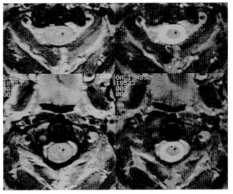

A   B

FIGURE 10.4 Hematomyelia.
Follow-up at 6 months in a patient who presented with sudden quadriplegia, Horner syndrome, and impaired deglutition and equilibrium. Persistence of lingual atrophy and left hemiplegia. T1 spin echo coronal (**A**) and T2 axial (**B**) sequences show a linear bulbomedullar hyposignal (→) lateralized to the left, suggesting old bleeding (hemosiderin). After arteriography, a diagnosis of bleeding telangiectasia was made.

Lesions in the Subarachnoid Pathway

Clinical Aspects

There are no specific clinical aspects regarding lesions in the subarachnoid pathway. A lesion to the XII nerve can be isolated. The proximity of the vertebral artery explains the frequency of vascular causes.

Etiologies

- Tumors
  - Primary tumors in the nerve (neurinoma) (Fig. 10.5)
  - Local compression (meningioma, metastasis)
- Vascular causes
  - Aneurysm of the vertebral artery or arterial ectasia
  - Meningeal hemorrhage (hemosiderin)
- Infectious causes
  - Meningitis of the base of the skull (tuberculosis)

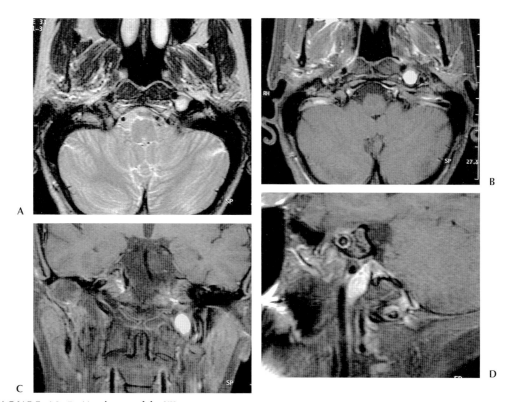

FIGURE 10.5 Neurinoma of the XII nerve.
Left paralysis of XII nerve. Oval mass extending from the hypoglossal foramen to the retrostyloid space in hypersignal T2 and marked enhancement. **(A)** T2 axial sequence. **(B–D)** T1 sequences after gadolinium injection.

- The craniovertebral junction
  - Subdislocation (rheumatoid arthritis)
  - Chiari malformation

At the Hypoglossal Canal

Clinical Aspects

A lesion in the XII nerve at the hypoglossal canal can be isolated. The most frequent cause is metastasis to the occipital bone that requires exploration of the osseous window of the base of the skull.

Etiologies

- Tumors
  - Primary tumors (meningioma, chordoma) or secondary to the occipital bone (lung, breast, prostate, pelvis via Batson plexus) (Fig. 10.6)
  - Spread from a nasopharyngeal tumor
  - Jugular glomus tumor

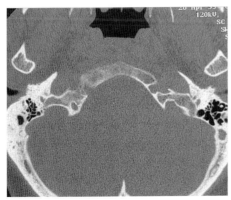
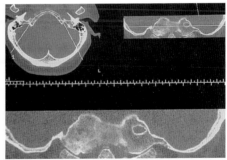

FIGURE 10.6   Occipital metastasis.
The patient was examined for an adenocarcinoma of the prostate. Right paralysis of the XII nerve. Axial section and curvilinear reconstruction with a bone window. Condensing lesion in the clivus, centered on the hypoglossal canal with lysis of cortical bone compatible with metastasis (→). The retrostyloid syndrome consists of paralysis of the IX, X, XI, and XII nerves, as well as paralysis of the cervical sympathetic nerves (Horner syndrome).

- Bone-related causes, including malformations of the junction and occipital fracture (Fig. 10.7)
- Infectious causes, including osteomyelitis of the skull base
- Other causes, including Paget disease and fibrous dysplasia

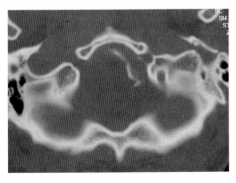

FIGURE 10.7   Occipital fracture after head trauma.
Paralysis of the left velum palati and the left half of the tongue. Axial bone section showing the fracture–dislocation of the left occipital condyle with a displaced bone fragment near the foramen magnum (→).

In the Peripheral Pathway

Clinical Aspects

The condylojugular syndrome or Collet-Sicard syndrome is constituted by lesions in the IX, X, XI, and XII nerves.

The XII nerve can be injured very distally in the retrostyloid space, in the hyoid area, opposite the loop in XII nerve, or even along the lingual pathway and in the sublingual space.

Etiologies

In The Retrostyloid, Nasopharyngeal, And Oropharyngeal Spaces.

- Tumors
    - Spread from a pharyngeal tumor (Fig. 10.8)

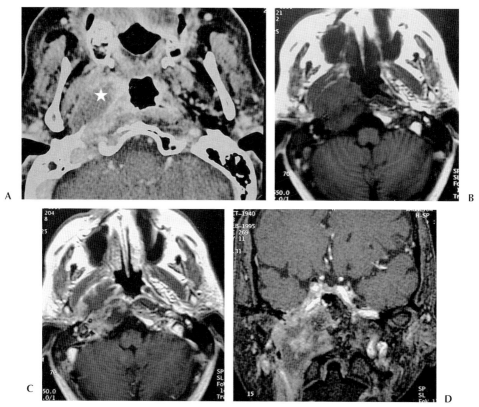

FIGURE 10.8 Carcinoma of the tonsil.

A 55-year-old patient with right ear pain, neck discomfort, and right paralysis of the XII nerve. Expanding process in the right paratonsillar area (★), the medial pterygoid muscle, the carotid space contacting the jugular foramen, and the prevertebral space. There is a bone lesion in the right baso-occipital area with disappearance of the T1 fat signal (**C**). Right serous otitis (**B**). In the coronal sequence, there is intracranial extension to the trigeminal cavum, the cavernous sinus, and the peritemporal meninges (**D**). (**A**) Computed axial tomographic scan section with injection. (**B**) T1 axial spin echo sequence. (**C**) T1 axial spin echo sequence with contrast injection. (**D**) Coronal T1 spin echo sequence with fat suppressed and contrast injection.

- Malignant tumor of the accessory salivary glands or the parotid gland
- Lymph node metastasis
- Lymphoma
- Neurinoma of the mixed nerves (Fig. 10.3)
- Lipoma
- Paraganglioma
- Infiltration of a nerve (amylosis) (Fig. 10.9)
- Vascular causes
  - Dissection of the internal carotid
  - Carotid aneurysm
  - Thrombophlebitis of the internal jugular vein

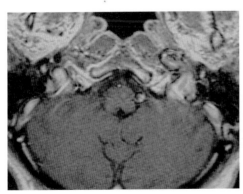
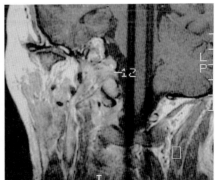

A   B

FIGURE 10.9 **Amyloid neuropathy present for 8 years in a 68-year-old patient.**
Sensory impairment of the lower limbs and asymmetric lingual atrophy. **(A)** Axial T1 spin echo sequence after injection.
(B) Parasagittal oblique T1 sequence with injection. The XII nerve appears enlarged and swollen along the pathway in the
foramen and the retrostyloid space (→).

- Infectious causes
  - Spread from an abscess in the retropharyngeal, parotid, and/or prevertebral spaces
- Iatrogenic causes
  - Radiotherapy
  - Needle entry into the jugular vein
  - Complication from an endarteriotomy

Tongue and Sublingual Space

- Malignant tumor of the base of the tongue and the floor of the mouth
- Infection in the sublingual space (of dental origin)
- Iatrogenic: dental extraction of a wisdom tooth, tonsillectomy

Vascularization of the Cranial Nerves

D. Doyon and A. Chays

ANATOMY

Vascular disorders play an important role in the pathogenesis of neuralgias and cranial nerve paralysis; they probably cause a percentage of the numerous "essential" neuralgias or a frigore paralysis encountered. Libersa and Lasjaunias have described the vascularization of the cranial nerves; besides the vertebrobasilar and internal carotid systems, which branch off into thin ramifications, the middle meningeal and accessory arteries vascularize the V2, V3, and VII nerves (also vascularized by the stylomastoid) (Fig. 11.1).

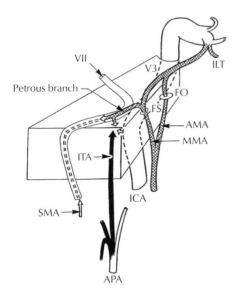

FIGURE 11.1 Diagram representing the middle meningeal system at the base of the skull.
The middle meningeal (MMA) and accessory meningeal arteries (AMA) contribute to the vascularization of the V3 nerve. There are anastomoses with the posterior branch of the inferolateral trunk (ILT) through the oval foramen (FO) and the foramen spinosum (FS). The petrosal branch of the middle meningeal artery vascularizes the VII nerve in the facial canal, where it anastomoses with the inferior tympanic artery (ITA), coming from the ascending pharyngeal artery (APA) and the stylomastoid artery (SMA) branch of the posterior auricular artery. ICA, internal carotid artery. From Lapresle J, Lasjaunias P. Cranial nerve ischemic arterial syndromes. A review. *Brain* 109:207–216, 1996. Reproduced with the authorization of Oxford University Press.

The inferolateral trunk of the carotid siphon vascularizes the V1 nerve and the III, IV and VI nerves (Fig. 11.2). The ascending pharyngeal artery vascularizes the IX, X, XI, and XII nerves (see Figs. 9.10 and 11.3). The middle meningeal and accessory arteries, the inferolateral trunk of the carotid siphon and the ascending pharyngeal artery have abundant anastomoses.

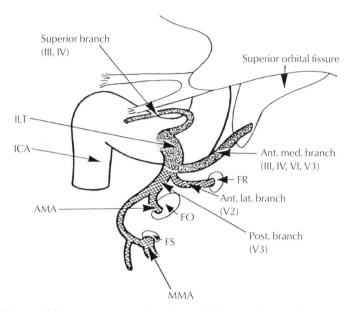

FIGURE 11.2 Diagram of the intracavernous internal carotid (ICA) and the inferolateral trunk (ILT) coming from the horizontal portion of the carotid siphon, which vascularizes the II and IV nerves.

The anteromedial branch penetrates into the orbit through the superior orbital fissure and vascularizes the III, IV, VI ,and V1 nerves. The anterolateral branch travels to the round foramen and vascularizes the V2 nerve. The posterior branch vascularizes the V3 nerve (both motor and sensory). In addition, there are anastomoses between the cavernous branches, the accessory meningeal arteries (AMA), and the middle meningeal arteries (MMA). FO, foramen ovale; FS, foramen spinosum. From Lapresle J, Lasjaunias P. Cranial nerve ischemic arterial syndromes. A review. *Brain* 1986; 109:207–215. Reproduced with the authorization of the Oxford University Press.

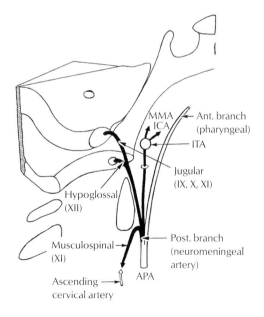

FIGURE 11.3 Diagram representing the ascending pharyngeal artery system (APS) at the posterior portion of the base of the skull, lateral view.

The ascending pharyngeal artery (APA) branches off to the three main trunks: anterior (ant. branch); the inferior tympanic artery (ITA), which anastomoses with the middle meningeal artery (MMA) and the internal carotid (ICA); and the posterior branch (post. branch). The ascending pharyngeal artery then branches off into three subdivisions that vascularize the most caudate nerves: the jugular branch for the IX, X, and XI nerves; the hypoglossal branch for the XII nerves; and the musculospinal branch for the XI nerve. Below and behind, the musculospinal artery anastomoses with the ascending cervical artery, which vascularizes the cervical nerves from C3 to C6. From Lapresle J, Lasjaunias P. Cranial nerve ischemic arterial syndromes. A review. *Brain* 109:207–216, 1986. Reproduced with the authorization of the Oxford University Press.

PHYSIOPATHOLOGY

Ischemic vascular lesions of the cranial nerves can be seen in arterial hypertension, diabetes mellitus, arteritis (viral or other), or trauma. Ischemic vascular lesions are also sometimes related to dissections, an arteriovenous fistula, or to selective embolization of the above-mentioned branches.

Although embolization has provided a description of arterial vascular territories, the clinical presentation sometimes provides the proof when there is simultaneous impairment in the facial and the V nerves in a frigore facial paralysis; the vascularization of the V and VII nerves is provided by the middle meningeal and accessory meningeal arteries. (The I, II, and VIII nerves are not true cranial nerves and have a special vascularization.)

VASCULAR LOOPS

"Vascular loops" must be considered separately. Vascular loops can enter into conflict with the cranial nerves at the level of the arteries of the base of the skull or compress or directly distort the brainstem near the area where they enter or exit.

Although the pathophysiogenesis of nerve or nerve nuclei damage from conflict or compression has not yet been clearly demonstrated, it is generally accepted that

- The transition zone between central myelin (constituted by oligodendrocytes) and peripheral myelin (formed by Schwann cells) is a zone that is particularly sensitive and exposed to the conflict. This transition zone is commonly called *the root entry zone* (REZ).
- Although vascular loops are numerous in the cisterns of the base of the skull and, consequently, artery-to-nerve contacts frequent, only a few anatomic predispositions that have been well identified can explain the clinical expression of a conflict.

It appears that all of the nerves can be involved. Conflicts with the facial nerve (VII) produce hemifacial spasm and those involving the trigeminal nerve (V) can elicit facial neuralgia (Trousseau neuralgia). Vascular compression involving the mixed nerves (particularly the IX nerve) and the oculomotor nerves are next in frequency and the acoustic nerve is only rarely subjected to compression by a vascular loop.

This can be explained by the anatomic study of the relationship between the vertebrobasilar arterial system and the mixed nerves, the acousticofacial and the trigeminal. Despite the fact that the localizations, pathways, and endings of these blood vessels are very variable from one side of the body to the other in the same subject and from one individual to another, memorization of the schematic representation can allow the clinician to explain all situations encountered (Fig. 11.4).

The vertebral arteries, ideally symmetrical, unite to form a basilar artery, which is generally median. The posteroinferior cerebellar arteries (PICA) originate from the vertebral arteries. The anteroinferior (AICA) and anterosuperior (ACS) cerebellar arteries originate from the basilar trunk.

It is easy to imagine an infinite number of anatomic variations in these arteries, with the most frequent being asymmetry in the two vertebral arteries, one of which is hypoplasic and the other is voluminous and climbs high in the cerebellopontine angle. This voluminous vertebral artery pushes the PICA upward and toward the back, thereby creating a conflict with the VII nerve in its penetration zone into the brainstem, representing the most frequent cause of hemifacial spasm. In addition to arteries, the presence of veins can add to the conflict; a nerve can be pinched between an artery and a vein or, more rarely, by the direct compression of a venous segment. According to the nerve, the arteries involved vary (Fig. 11.5).

Arterial conflicts between the VII nerve, clinically inducing hemifacial spasm, can be due to the following (see Figs. 7.17 and 11.6): a vertebral artery, especially at its ending, where it forms the

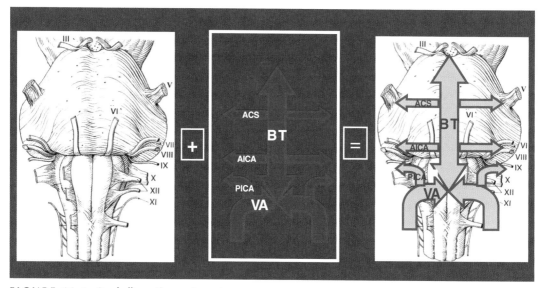

FIGURE 11.4 Cerebellopontine angle anatomy.
A perfectly symmetrical vertebrobasilar artery (VA = vertebral artery) system. Relationships between the cranial nerves
(VII, VIII, III and V) (BT = basilar artery).

basilar trunk with the contralateral artery; a PICA; an AICA; or the association between the two, or
even three, arteries.

Hemifacial spasm is a clinical entity involving the sudden, involuntary, painless, and unilateral
contraction of the facial muscles. This peripheral motor phenomenon successively goes through
clonic, tonic-clonic, and, finally, tonic phases. The cause had long remained undetermined and the
syndrome was termed "essential"; today, it is explained by the existence of a neurovascular conflict
at the facial nerve's exit point at the REZ, the nerve's entrance or exit zone that is located a few
millimeters from the brainstem. The particular anatomic variation involving a voluminous vertebral
artery that climbs high in the cerebellopontine angle predisposes to the appearance of a spasm
over time. Arterial hypertension also appears to play a role in the formation of arterial loops.

Vascular conflicts in the V nerve produce trigeminal neuralgia (see Fig. 6.10) and are related
to a superior cerebellar artery (SCA) in nearly three quarters of cases. They also involve a cerebellar vein in 25% of cases. Neurovascular conflicts of the VIII nerve elicit tinnitus and/or vertigo. The
AICA is the vessel most often responsible, followed by the PICA and the association of a vertebral
artery to the PICA. Neurovascular conflicts involving the IX nerve produce so-called essential glos-
sodynia, a rare phenomenon. It is caused by the vertebral artery or sometimes by an association
between a vertebral artery and a PICA (see Fig. 9.8). Table 11.1 reports a series of conflicts that
were surgically explored and provides the statistical distribution of the responsible vessels.

As a reminder, the diagnostic radiographic criteria for neurovascular conflicts are as follows:

- Vascular contact with the nerve root (in its REZ)
- A vessel that is perpendicular to the nerve's pathway
- Deviation or distortion of the nervous structures

With recent developments in radiologic techniques, blood vessels and nerves can be clearly
visualized on the same radiographic film, allowing the radiologist to study the vessel's pathway, the
site of conflict, eventual nerve distortion, and the adjacent nerve structures.

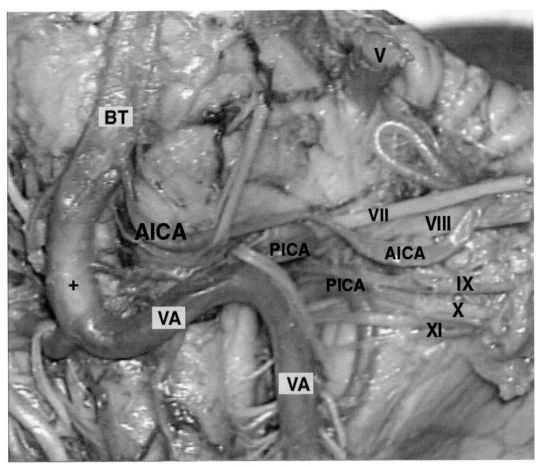

FIGURE 11.5   Endoscopic view of the left cerebellopontine cistern.
Note hypertrophy in the left vertebral artery (VA) which pushes the posteroinferior cerebellar artery against the VII nerve.

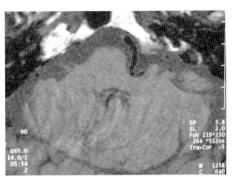

FIGURE 11.6   Left hemifacial spasm.
Loop in the left posteroinferior cerebellar artery pushing the point of origin of the left VII nerve and leaving an imprint on its exit point from the pons thin axial section during T1 sequence.

MR image should include high-resolution (constructive interference in steady state, three-dimensional fast spin echo) T2-weighted sequences that are capable of clearly defining the neurovascular relationships, as well as angiomagnetic resonance sequences with an analysis of native

TABLE 11.1 Statistical Table of Vascular Loops Explaining a Number of Cases of Cranial Nerve Involvement

	Hemifacial Spasm	Trigeminal Neuralgia	Tinnitus
Isolated AICA	13		60
Isolated PICA	16		27
Isolated vertebral artery	7		
Vertebral artery + PICA	45		13
Vertebral artery + PICA + AICA	8		
Vein + AICA	4		
Vein + PICA	4		
Vein + superior cerebellar artery		29	
Isolated vein	0.5	21	
Isolated superior cerebellar artery		50	

Values are expressed as percentages.
Data compiled by J. Magnan et al.
AICA indicates anteroinferior cerebellar artery; PICA, posteroinferior cerebellar artery.

slices and reconstructions. A supratentorial fluid-attenuated inversion recovery T2 sequence as well as T1 sequences with and without the injection of contrast material are indispensable to exclude demyelinating or intra-axial disease or a tumor along the nerve's pathway. With modern techniques, the radiologist is capable of studying the conflict site, its range, the responsible vessels, and the eventual distortion of the neighboring nervous structures (see Fig. 7.17).

The clinical and imaging findings can help in the decision of the surgical indication, the intent of which is to remove the conflict(s) and interpose a Teflon (DuPont, Wilmington, DE, USA) fragment between the nerve and the vessel. Surgery should be performed as soon as the imaging confirms the clinical diagnosis. After decompression, cure is obtained in 95% of cases of spasm and in nearly 80% of cases of Trousseau neuralgia.

CONCLUSION

In conclusion, a comparison between clinical and imaging findings often provides a precise diagnosis in cranial nerve disorders but there are still some so-called essential or a frigore neuralgias. A vascular cause including dissecting aneurysm, arterial hypertension, diabetes mellitus, or vascular loops should not be overlooked.

Functional MRI of the Brain and the Functional Analysis of the Cranial Nerves

D. Ducreux

Functional MR image (fMRI) is an expanding imaging technique that allows the examination of the the brain functions allotted to a given situation in a completely innocuous manner. It is routinely used clinically during the presurgical workup for brain tumors to pinpoint the central sulcus and the primary motor areas or to assess language lateralization, but it can also be useful in analyzing at the cortical or subcortical level certain sensory integration functions such as vision, audition, smell, or taste.

PHYSICAL PRINCIPLES

The principle of fMRI is based on an observation during the past century (an observation that has since been verified by Weisskoff): regions activated during any cerebral task have a transitory increase in their corresponding cerebral blood flow (with an increase in vessel size) and increased local metabolism.

Coupling of cerebral activation–perfusion shows paradoxical blood oxygenation in the venulae supplying the activated area. The increase in oxygen consumption in the activated regions is quantitatively lower than the supply.

Use of the magnetic properties of hemoglobin in different oxygenation states has given rise to the blood oxygenation level–dependent (BOLD) contrast, which is principally used in fMRI: oxyhemoglobin, which is diamagnetic, does not produce any change in the local magnetic field, whereas desoxyhemoglobin, which is paramagnetic, does produce change in the local magnetic field.

Thus, desoxyhemoglobin induces a reduction in the magnitude of the signal obtained from an MRI sequence capable of magnetic sensitivity (such as gradient-echo or echoplanar sequences).

It is the oxyhemoglobin (very augmented)-to-desoxyhemoglobin (relatively stable) ratio that induces a paradoxical hypersignal (because in the activated area the quantity of paramagnetic substance induces less of a reduction than in nonactivated areas). This hypersignal is weak (a small percentage at most) and depends on the strength of the magnetic field (undetectable at 1 tesla [T], it varies between 1 and 5% at 1.5 T and attains approximately 15% at 3 T).

Thus, fMRI is a tool that can be used to measure the qualitative variations in local blood oxygenation, mainly in the venulae. Variations in the temporal resolution—approximately a few seconds and sometimes a few tenths of a second in a very strong field—correspond to an early signal fall (**early deep**) due to the production of desoxyhemoglobin. These resolutions are very slow compared with neuron conduction velocities. Spatial resolution varies by a few millimeters. Resolution increases according to the intensity of the magnetic field by an increase in the signal-to-sound ratio.

Certain artifacts such as physiologic noise (heart beats or respiratory sounds) or artifacts contained in the sequences used (distortions during echoplanar sequences, notably in temporal or frontal air–bone–tissue interface areas) increase with the intensity of the field and can artificially create or erase the activated zones. Nevertheless, one can compensate for these artifacts by using image-correcting algorithms or by subtracting the physiologic noise. There is a tendency to prefer experimental neurocognitive studies using very strong fields (>3 T) and clinical studies using 1.5 T MRI, which is actually the most widely used.

SIGNAL ANALYSIS

Because the percent of the signal increase in activated cerebral areas is weak at 1.5 T and the temporal resolution of the BOLD contrast study is limited to a few seconds (early deep signal analysis is impossible), it is difficult to identify the activated cerebral areas implicated during rapidly fluctuating phenomenon. Thus, only relatively simple, repetitive tasks of sufficient duration that are adapted to the study can be assessed. Accordingly, **paradigms** have been created corresponding to the temporal arrangement of tasks that the subject must effect (generally alternating action phases with rest periods for en bloc paradigms). Certain refinements can be employed to study time-limited events: event fMRI.

Thus, fMRI corresponds to an analysis of the temporal variations in signal as a function of a given paradigm. Because of the above-mentioned limitations, this analysis can only be used to demonstrate a significant difference existing between two states (eg, activation and rest) by subtracting series of images and by refining the results through the use of statistical t and F tests, and by calculating z scores or correlation coefficients (actually the most commonly used).[1] This analysis is subject to multiple artifacts, with the most troublesome being artifacts due to movement, which require that the subject remain perfectly immobile during the entire study. Similarly, artifacts from persistent activation, notably during memory or olfactory stimulation, pose a real methodologic problem because the rest phase is difficult to define.

Once the calculations are made, two- or three-dimensional stereotactic activation cartographies can be obtained by superimposing the statistical probability cartographies onto the anatomic acquisitions (Fig. 12.1).

fMRI is useful in studying both simple neurologic functions and more complex cognitive functions. Interpretation of fMRI requires not only perfect knowledge of MRI techniques but also a sound understanding of certain fundamental neurophysiologic concepts. We will limit the remainder of this chapter to a few current investigations, notably fMRI of vision (eye jerks [ocular pursuit movements] included) and of audition, and we will mention some existing data relative to the senses of smell and taste (Figs. 12.2 to 12.4).

1. Bandettini PA, Jesmanowicz A, Wong EC, Hyde JS. Processing strategies for time-course data sets in functional MRI of the human brain. *Magn Reson Med* 1993;30: 161–173.

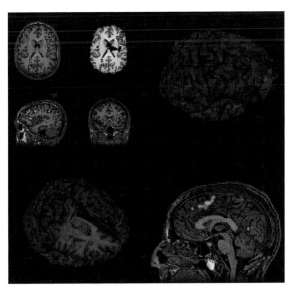

FIGURE 12.1   Activation cartography during category verbal fluency test.
Projection of the coded activations according to a color scale during a spoiled gradient recalled acquisition in steady state (SPGR) T1-weighted volumetric sequence with multiplane (above and on the left) and sagittal (below and on the right) views. Corresponding three-dimensional surface reconstructions with stereotactic projections of the activations. The activation foci are located near the cingular cortex, the dorsolateral prefrontal cortex, and the insula.

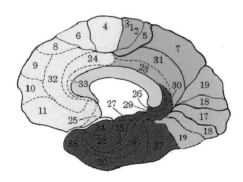

FIGURE 12.2   Diagram of some of the Brodmann areas.
Medial cerebral surface. Motor, premotor, and prefrontal (yellow) areas and sensory and associative (green) and visual (blue) areas are shown.

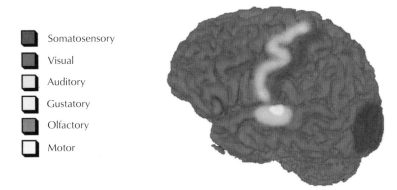

Somatosensory

Visual

Auditory

Gustatory

Olfactory

Motor

FIGURE 12.3   Three-dimensional surface reconstruction of a brain acquired with a T1-weighted volumetric sequence.
Right posterolateral view. The different color codes represent projections from the corresponding areas.

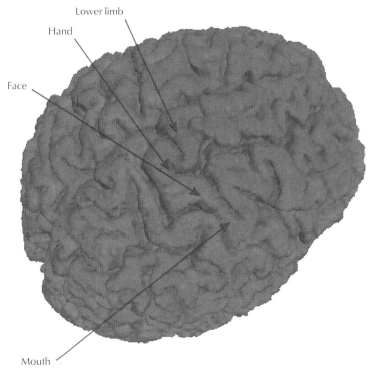

Lower limb

Hand

Face

Mouth

FIGURE 12.4 **Somatotopic organization of the sensorimotor cortex.**
Three-dimensional surface brain reconstruction acquired with a T1-weighted volumetric sequence. Left superolateral view. The cortical areas corresponding to the lower limbs are higher and more medial compared with the areas corresponding to the upper limbs and the face.

VISUAL SYSTEM

Functional Neuroanatomy

The axon leaves the retina by the intermediary of the optic nerve (Figs. 12.3 to 12.6). The optic nerve travels to the optic chiasma, where a portion of its fibers cross (the nasal portion) and the remaining fibers (temporal portion) receive the contralateral contingent and form the optic tract. The optic tract surrounds the cerebral peduncles and travels toward the lateral genicular nucleus (LGN); the remaining axons travel toward the superior colliculus and the pretectal lamina (Fig. 12.5).

The neurons of the LGN send their axons directly to the primary visual cortex (V1) by means of the optic radiations through the temporal and parietal white matter. Accordingly, specialized neuron **clusters** (groups of similar P and M neurons dedicated to a function) are organized from the retina to the visual cortex. The visual functions are segmented into different categories: eg, color vision, line vision, movement vision. The visual parietal cortex (MT and PP) appears to be implicated in movement vision and spatial orientation, and the temporal visual cortex (V4 and IT) seems more connected to the complex process of object recognition. Emotional reactions are associated with the temporal amygdala.

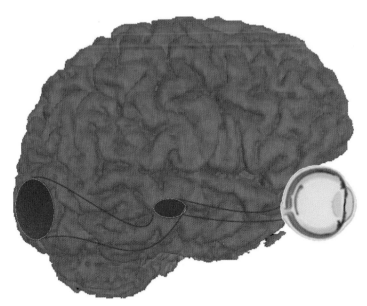

FIGURE 12.5   Morphofunctional diagram of vision.
Three-dimensional surface brain reconstruction acquired by a T1-weighted volumetric sequence. Left lateral view. The visual cortex is the projection area for fibers coming from the superior colliculus, whose fibers have come from the optic nerves.

Functional MRI

The first brain activations, obtained by simple luminous stimulations coming from a flash, demonstrated cortical clusters in the territory of the primary visual area (AB 17, V1) (Fig. 12.6). The bilateral associative visual areas are activated in the occipital lobe by a more complex or wider stimulation (AB 18 and 19). The striate visual areas (AB 17 or V1) or extrastriated areas (AB 18 and 19, or V2, VP, V3, and V4) present a retinotopic organization, an aid for central vision that is more striking than that in nonhuman primates.

The study of jerking eye movements, performed with positron emission tomography (PET) and later with MRI, has helped to localize the specific cortical areas implicated: frontal (AB 8, 6, 4, and 9) and parietal (AB 39 and 40) areas. In the same way, certain midtemporal areas (AB 19, 37, and 39) activate in the same manner during ocular pursuit.

By using specific visual stimulations, the cortical areas that are sensitive to forms and contours have been located. Similarly, certain areas sensitive to movement and color variations are simultaneously activated; this has helped to establish a relationship between the perception of movement (area MT), contrast, and light intensity.

During mental recall of a visual stimulus effected in previous experiments and in the absence of any concomitant stimulation, activation foci in the primary visual cortex have been identified. This **mental imagery**, which is actually used to study the motor cortex and the language areas, may constitute an important avenue for exploring certain disorders that prevent patients from active participation in motor or language activities.

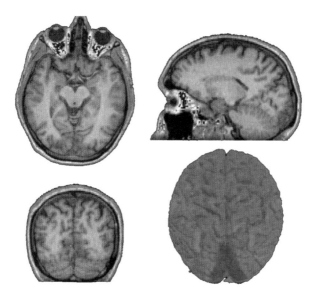

FIGURE 12.6 Functional MR image by visual stimulation.
First experiment. Activations located in the primary visual cortex (in red) are seen on these axial, sagittal, coronal, and three-dimensional surface reconstructions.

AUDITORY SYSTEM

Functional Neuroanatomy

Information from sounds emitted from the cochlea arrives at the brainstem (cochlear nucleus) by the acoustic (VIII) nerve (Fig. 12.7). After reaching the brainstem, the fibers separate and some of them travel toward the ipsilateral and contralateral ventral cochlear nuclei, then toward the superior olivae. There, a first analysis of the signal is performed to determine the direction of the sound (by using temporal comparison of the afferents). The superior oliva then projects toward the inferior colliculus by the lateral lemniscus. A second stream of information leaves the dorsal cochlear nucleus, which performs a spectral sound analysis (frequencies) and travels toward the two inferior colliculi (ipsilateral and contralateral) through the lateral lemniscus.

The fibers from the two inferior colliculi travel toward the ipsilateral medial geniculate nucleus, which in turn projects toward the primary auditory cortex (Heschl superior temporal gyrus, AB 41).

There is great individual variation in the distribution of auditory fibers and their corresponding projections. Nevertheless, it appears that the tonotopic organization (Fig. 12.8) of the fibers used to transport high-frequency information is located medially and produces a lateralization of auditory functions. Accordingly, the left temporal lobe probably treats language information better, whereas the right temporal lobe is concerned with natural sounds.

Functional MRI

Because of noise, the MRI sequences used in auditory fMRI can constitute a parasitic auditory stimulation, the characteristics of which (eg, intensity, frequency, duration, the fact that subjects become accustomed to it, various emotional or cognitive reactions such as fear) are difficult to control (Fig. 12.9). Similarly, complete rest periods are difficult to achieve during particularly noisy

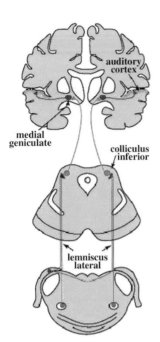

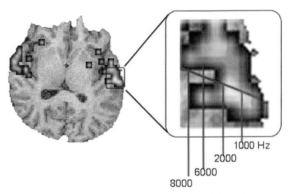

FIGURE 12.7   Diagram of the auditory tracts.
The fibers from the cochlear nuclei relay with the superior oliva and project toward the inferior colliculus via the lateral lemniscus, then travel toward the primary auditory cortex in Heschl superior temporal gyrus.

FIGURE 12.8   Tonotopic organization of the primary auditory cortex.
Activation cartography obtained after bilateral auditory stimulation. The integration of the auditory information follows a frequency organization, with high frequencies treated medially as compared with low frequencies.

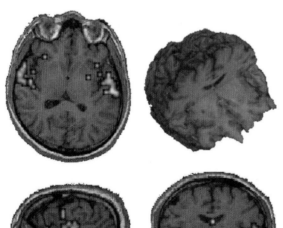

FIGURE 12.9   Activation cartography, auditory stimulation test.
Projection of coded activations according to a color scale during a spoiled gradient recalled acquisition in steady state T1-weighted volumetric sequence using multiplane views. Corresponding three-dimensional surface reconstructions with stereotactic projections of the activations. The activation foci are located in the white matter of the superior temporal cortex (Hesch┃

conditions (100 dB at 500 Hz).[2] Accordingly, to ensure the efficacy of sound stimulations, a sound must be emitted 30 dB above the parasite noise threshold; this may limit studies and may require various technical exploits (silent sequences).

Thus, the auditory system is explored by using verbal stimulations (comprehensible or incomprehensible languages or syllables) or by using sound stimulations after assessing the subjective auditory thresholds in the functioning apparatus. Stimulations like these can evoke the bilateral activations in the superior temporal gyrus (Heschl, AB 41 and 42) that maintain their tonotopic organization. These activations appear symmetric during pure tonal stimulations and asymmetric during semantic stimulations (middle temporal gyrus). In addition, left lateralization in certain right-handed subjects has been observed.

At 1.5 T, it is difficult to demonstrate activation **clusters** in the brainstem, the colliculi, or the geniculi nuclei because of the technical constraints related to the conditions of activation and insufficient spatial resolution. Nonetheless, studies using a very strong field (3 T or more) have objectively demonstrated pathologic focal lesions, notably in dyslexic (geniculi nucleus) or autistic (brainstem) patients.

VESTIBULAR SYSTEM

Functional Neuroanatomy

The vestibular nuclei (lateral, sense of balance, caudal, medial, rostral) receive afferents from the vestibule by the intermediary of the VIII nerve. The vestibular nuclei constitute the converging point for an array of sensorial (eg, rotation, translation, acceleration) and proprioceptive information after the influx from the vestibulospinal tractus, which provides the proprioceptive proprieties of the muscles of the neck and the cervical spine. The vestibular nuclei coordinate posture (posture reflex) and compensate for ocular movements (vestibulo-ocular reflex: helping to maintain the retinal image) and changes in the position of the head and the body (vestibulospinal reflex). Afterward, the influx travels toward the thalamus and then toward the vestibular cortex (near the somatosensory cortex).

Functional MRI

The vestibular system is stimulated by injecting cold water into the external auditory meatus (Fig. 12.10). Data are acquired when nystagmus induced by the stimulation ceases. Contralateral activations in areas AB 39, 40, 41, 42, and in the parietoinsular cortex (which is also seen during jerking eye movements [AB 39 and 40]) have been demonstrated. Similarly, ipsilateral activations in the putamen, area AB 7, the posterior portion of the cingular cortex, and the hippocampus have been demonstrated.

GUSTATORY SYSTEM

Functional Neuroanatomy

There are five primary gustatory senses: sweet, salty, meat, bitter, and acid (Fig. 12.11). The axons implicated in the sense of taste originate in the papillary cells of the tongue and the rhinopharyngeal mucosa. Gustatory thresholds depend on the temperature, the localization of the perception (tongue),

---

2. Cho ZH, Chung SC, Lim DW, Wong EK. Effects of the acoustic noise of the gradient systems on fMRI: A study on auditory, motor, and visual cortices. *Magn Reson Med* 1998; 39: 331–335.

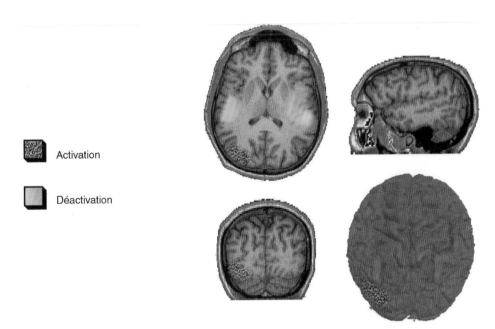

FIGURE 12.10 Functional MR image.
Activation cartography during right vestibular cold tests. The parietoinsular activation foci (in green) and the posterior parietal deactivation (in orange) illustrate the complex cerebral control in the vestibular reflex.

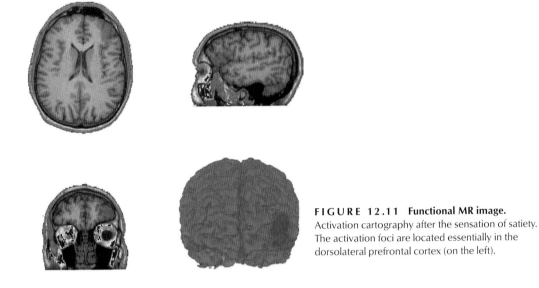

FIGURE 12.11 Functional MR image.
Activation cartography after the sensation of satiety. The activation foci are located essentially in the dorsolateral prefrontal cortex (on the left).

and the age and genetic composition of the subject. Adaptation and potential maximization phenomena are present after exposure to certain tastes (eg, bitter and sweet, sweet and salty). Similarly, there are latency phenomena after exposure. The conduction pathways originate directly in the cells of the tongue (they do not cross), are transported by the chorda tympani (VII) nerve and the glossopharyngeal (IX) nerve to the solitary nucleus, which projects toward the ventral and posteromedial thalamic nuclei, then toward the somatosensorial cortex in the area of the mouth and the vomit centers (brainstem).

OLFACTORY SYSTEM

Functional Neuroanatomy

The olfactory receptors project their fibers through the cribriform lamina of the ethmoid via the intermediary of the olfactory tracts toward the paleocortex (dorsomedial thalamic nucleus), which is associated with the limbic system and is thus implicated in emotions and memories (amygdala, hippocampus). The fibers then travel toward the orbitofrontal olfactory neocortex and the hypothalamus (a vomeronasal organ that has a hormonal influence on olfactory perceptions) (Fig. 12.12). Detection of the direction of an odor influx is influenced by an inhibition influx, which is situated between the two olfactory bulbs and is carried by the anterior commissure.

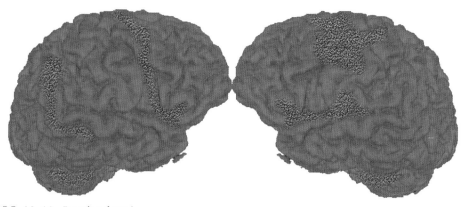

FIGURE 12.12 Functional MR image.
Three-dimensional surface activation cartography obtained after odorous stimulations. The activation foci are situated in the olfactory areas and in the parietal, prefrontal, and cerebellar cortices.

CONCLUSION

The cranial nerves can be viewed as conduction systems between peripheral sensory organs and the receptor, the cerebral cortex, or the muscular response. Future progress in fMRI brought about by refinements in cortical analysis will provide a clearer picture of the relays in these information-transmitting pathways (eg, colliculus, nuclei of the pons). Accordingly, a book dedicated to the cranial nerves must mention the anatomic transmission pathways as well as their integration centers, which are easily assessed by this imaging technique.

13

The Sympathetic and Parasympathetic Nervous Systems of the Head and Neck

J. -L. Sarrazin, P. de Greslan, and J. -L. Poncet

The autonomic nervous system ensures the regulation of vegetative functions. It controls the motility of the viscera, the glands, the blood vessels, and nonstriate muscles (Figs. IX–XII).

Two distinct parts can be distinguished in its anatomy and function: the sympathetic system and the parasympathetic system. At the cephalic extremity of the system, in addition to vasoregulation, the two systems provide innervation to the intrinsic eye muscles and regulate the secretions of the lacrimal and salivary glands. The nerves of the parasympathetic system are intimately connected to certain cranial nerves, thereby explaining some of the signs encountered during the course of lesions in cranial nerves. The sympathetic nerves are more related to blood vessels; this may explain why lesions in the sympathetic nerves can express their own specific symptoms. The association of signs due to a lesion in the autonomic nervous system, with neurologic symptoms related to another cause, can help determine the precise location of the causal lesions. Consequently, a thorough knowledge of the anatomy and clinical aspects of the autonomic nervous system is particularly important.

ANATOMY

General Organization

The hypothalamus is the organization center for the entire autonomic nervous system (Figs. 13.1–13.3). Stimulation of the anterior hypothalamus produces excitation in the parasympathetic system, whereas stimulation in the posterior portion results in excitation in the sympathetic system. The medial tractus of the telencephalon, the mamillotegmental tractus, and the dorsal longitudinal tract connect it with the reticular substance of the diencephalon, which provides the central impulsions to the two systems, the sympathetic and the parasympathetic. The preganglion fibers originate in the nuclear centers; they relay in the ganglions, where the second neuron is situated. The fibers coming from this ganglion (postganglion fibers) innervate the target organs.

The Parasympathetic System

In the encephalic extremity, the parasympathetic nuclei are located in the brainstem and in the nuclei of the oculomotor (III), facial (VII), glossopharyngeal (IX), and vagus (X) nerves. The preganglion fibers are long, whereas the postganglion fibers are short and originate in the ganglion cells located near the target organs.

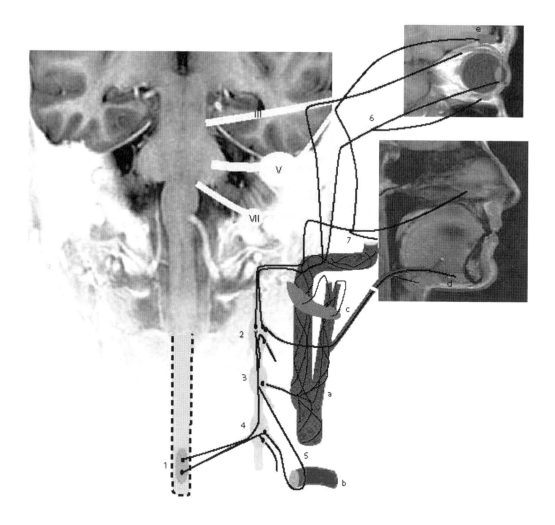

1. Medullar centrum	a. Carotid artery
2. Superior cervical	b. Subclavian artery
sympathetic ganglion	c. Parotid artery
3. Middle cervical	d. Submandibular gland
sympathetic ganglion	e. Lacrimal gland
4. Inferior cervical	
sympathetic ganglion	
5. Ansa cervicalis	
6. Ciliary ganglion	
7. Pterygopalatine ganglion	

FIGURE 13.1   Head and neck: The sympathetic system.

Parasympathetic Fibers Accompany the Oculomotor Nerve. The preganglion fibers are integrated into the motor fibers of the nerve. They leave the nerve at the superior orbital fissure and travel to the ciliary ganglion, where they synapse with the postganglion fibers that innervate the intrinsic eye muscles. Thus, a parasympathetic lesion results in

- Paralysis in the sphincter muscles of the pupil and, consequently, mydriasis
- Loss of the photomotor reflex
- Impaired convergence and accommodation

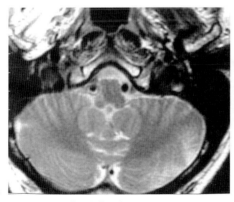
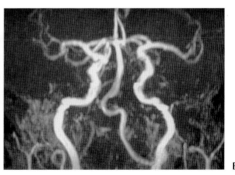

FIGURE 13.2   Bulbar infarction.
(A) T2-weighted axial section. (B) Angiomagnetic resonance during time of flight. Hyperintense lesion in the right lateral portion of the bulb in the retroolivary fossa. Absence of flux in the vertebral and right posteroinferior cerebellar artery. Wallenberg syndrome with Horner syndrome and alternate syndrome (paralysis of one half of the velum palati [of the hemipharynx], ipsilateral cerebellar syndrome, and hemiparesis of the contralateral extremities).

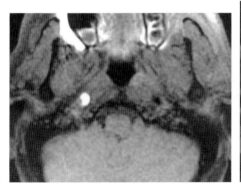
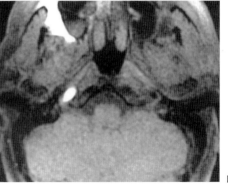

FIGURE 13.3   Internal carotid artery dissection.
(A,B) T1-weighted axial sections with saturation of the fat signal. Hematoma of the wall of the right internal carotid artery in its extracranial segment and in the right carotid canal, hyperintense appearance on these T1-weighted images. Carotid artery dissection with Horner syndrome and paralysis of the right 12th cranial pair.

Parasympathetic Fibers That Accompany the Facial Nerve. The efferent parasympathetic fibers form part of the intermediary nerve. The fibers originate in the superior salivary nucleus, which is located immediately beneath the motor nucleus of the VII nerve. A contingent of these fibers goes to the pterygopalatine ganglion to innervate the lacrimal glands and the glands of the nasal mucosa. Another group travels with the chorda tympani headed for the submandibular ganglion and provides innervation for the secretory function of the submandibular and sublingual glands.

Parasympathetic Fibers That Accompany the Glossopharyngeal and Vagus Nerves. Parasympathetic fibers originating in the inferior salivary nucleus travel in the tympanic nerve, a branch of the IX nerve, and relay in the otic ganglion to provide secretory innervation to the parotid gland. From the dorsal nucleus of the vagus nerve, the long preganglion fibers join with the different cephalic, thoracic, and abdominal ganglions before relaying in these postganglion fibers, thus providing innervation to the smooth muscles of the different viscera.

Sympathetic System

The centers of the sympathetic system that contain the preganglion fibers are situated in the lateral horns of the spinal cord. There is no center in the cervical spine and the sympathetic centers of the head and neck are located in the upper thoracic spine. The preganglion sympathetic fibers travel in the ventral root, then separate from the motoneurons in the spinal ganglion to form the white communicating ramification and join the sympathetic chain. The cervical sympathetic chain is composed of three ganglions:

- A superior ganglion
- A middle ganglion
- A cervicothoracic or stellate ganglion

The Superior Cervical Ganglion. The superior cervical ganglion is voluminous and fusiform; its superior pole is located approximately 2 cm beneath the carotid foramen and its inferior pole can be found at the C4 level. It is located in the retrostyloid space in front of the carotid artery and the internal jugular vein.

The Middle Cervical Ganglion. The middle cervical ganglion is inconstant but usually is located in front of the transversal process of C6.

The Stellate Ganglion. The stellate ganglion is located in the retropleural fossa, limited in front by the cervical pleura and in back by the transversal process of C7 and the neck of the first rib.

These three ganglions are linked together by anastomotic fibers. The postganglion fibers coming from these ganglions are not myelinated. The collateral branches of these ganglions are as follows:

- The sympathetic fibers coming from these ganglions that accompany the spinal nerves to the cutaneous dermatoma
- The sympathetic fibers that accompany the blood vessels and form plexuses that are intimately tied to these vessels destined for the effector organs. Special note should be made of the internal carotid nerve and the internal and external carotid plexuses, which come from the superior cervical ganglion.

The neurons for the nerves bound for the eye are located in the superior cervical ganglion. The postganglion fibers travel with the internal carotid nerve, then with the internal carotid plexus, and later accompany the oculomotor nerve headed for the levator palpebrae superioris muscle; the nasociliary nerve and the ciliary ganglion for the iris (pupil dilatation); the nerve of the pterygoid canal, the ptergyopalatine ganglion, the zygomatic branch of the maxillary nerve, and the lacrimal nerve intended for the lacrimal gland.

The superior and middle cervical ganglions contain the neurons of the nerves bound for the salivary glands. Their fibers travel in the external carotid plexus; then in the facial and lingual plexuses for the submandibular, sublingual, and lingual glands; and in the maxillary and temporal plexuses for the parotid gland.

The fibers bound for the sebaceous and sudoriferous glands of the head and neck originate in the three cervical ganglions. These fibers also provide sympathetic innervation to the arteries of the head and neck, particularly to the carotid arteries.

Clinical Aspects

Parasympathetic Lesions

Lesions to the parasympathetic system are never isolated: the preganglion fibers that are an integral part of the different cranial nerves cited previously are long, whereas the ganglions and the postganglion fibers are very close to the effector organs. Thus, the manifestations of parasympathetic lesions are contingent to the symptoms induced by the paralysis of a given cranial nerve:

- In lesions to the III nerve, in addition to the oculomotor impairment that predominates, pupil dilatation, loss of the photomotor reflex, and impaired accommodation are also seen.
- Lesions in the VII nerve produce facial paralysis plus, depending on its location, impaired secretion in the salivary (sublingual and submandibular glands) and lacrimal glands.
- Lesions in the IX and X nerves, may produce impaired salivary secretion (parotid gland).

Sympathetic Lesions

Inversely, sympathetic preganglion fibers are short and postganglion fibers are long and anatomically more individualized. They often travel in proximity to blood vessels. The most characteristic disorder in the cervical sympathetic system is Horner syndrome (HS), which in its complete form is defined by the unilateral association of the following clinical signs:

- Ptosis
- Myosis
- Enophthalmus
- Anhidrosis
- Vasodilatation of the hemiface

However, most often, a unilateral triad associating **ptosis, myosis,** and **enophthalmus** is encountered. A lesion in the sympathetic system, and more rarely a central lesion, causes this syndrome, most often in the cervical region.

Myosis corresponds to paralysis in the muscle that dilates the pupil; the result is predominance in the parasympathetic sphincter of the iris. One of the particularities of this myosis is the fact that pupil reactivity to light and to near-vision is conserved; accommodation is preserved.

Ptosis corresponds to closure of the palpebral fissure due to paralysis of the Müller muscle and of its homolog in the lower lid. This ptosis is not a paralytic ptosis. There is no increase in frontal action, and therefore, no eyebrow elevation.

There is no real *enophthalmus*. Actually, there is pseudoenopthalmus due to narrowing in the palpebral fissure aggravated by hypotonia of the smooth muscles.

Additional ocular signs have been described:

- Heterochromia of the iris
- Increase in the amplitude of accommodation
- Transitory ocular hypertonia
- Modifications in the retinal circulation
- Tearing
- Weak myopia

Horner syndrome is seen more often in its partial form than in its complete form, especially when accompanying brainstem lesions. The clinician should therefore remain particularly attentive during the patient physical examination and should suspect the syndrome whenever isolated ptosis or myosis is observed. HS can result from a lesion in the central neuron or in the preganglion or postganglion fibers.

Horner syndrome caused by a lesion in the central pathway involves the neuraxis (cerebral hemisphere, hypothalamus, brainstem, spinal cord). Thus, it is generally associated with other neurologic manifestations. **HS caused by a lesion in the preganglion** connecting the medullary center to the superior cervical ganglion is the segment involved, notably the first thoracic spinal nerve and the subclavian loop. Other causes include block from local anesthesia, a toxic effect from an injected fluid, overstretching, tumor, and neck surgery. **HS caused by a lesion in the postganglion** involves the third neuron connecting the superior cervical ganglion to the orbit.

The responsible lesion is most often extracranial. It can be due to a hematoma in the sheath of the carotid artery that compresses the small nutrient vessels of the superior cervical ganglion. The lesion may also occur during the course of certain cerebrovascular accidents caused by acute thrombosis of the internal carotid artery accompanied by pericarotid sympathetic involvement and resulting in an opticopyramidal syndrome associated with HS. The anatomy of the sympathetic system explains the numerous causes of HS. HS can result from a lesion in the brain or the spinal cord or from a cervical or cervicothoracic disorder.

Central Causes

Brain. HS can be due to a lesion in the brainstem, and particularly, the **medulla oblongata**. Vascular disorders are the most frequent causes (Babinski-Nageotte syndrome, Cestan-Chenais syndrome, Wallenberg syndrome). Very rarely, multiple sclerosis can cause HS.
Spinal Cord. A Chiari I malformation or syringomyelia can be accompanied by HS.

Cervical Causes

Cervical causes are the most frequent etiologies of HS.

Vascular Etiologies. Sympathetic fibers are intimately connected to arterial walls. In particular, the cervical sympathetic plexus and the internal carotid nerve accompany the internal carotid artery in its cervical segment and the first cranial segments (Fig. 13.1).

Agenesis of the internal carotid artery is unusual. HS can accompany it.

Carotid Dissection. A hematoma in the artery wall compresses the plexus and the internal carotid nerve; accordingly, HS is one of the major signs at the onset of dissection of the internal carotid artery (Fig. 13.2).

After Trauma or Vascular Surgery. Cervical tumors such as schwannomas or paragangliono-mas are rarely the cause of HS. Nevertheless, occasionally authentic schwannomas of the cervical sympathetic trunk can present clinically with HS.

Cervicothoracic Causes

Tumors in the cervicothoracic region are the most frequent causes of HS. The Pancoast-Tobias syndrome, which consists of a tumor in the apex of the lung, can be accompanied by HS. Certain forms of thyroiditis can also result in HS.

Diagnosis and Exploration

Most often, HS is part of **a patent, recognized neurologic syndrome.** In this case, the syndrome, when associated with other neurologic signs, can help **localize the lesion.** HS can also be **isolated** and occasionally **incomplete.** When that is the case, **an etiologic workup** is required, paying particular attention to the **mode of onset.**

Because HS can have a cerebral, medullary, or cervical cause, MR image is the most useful procedure for its exploration. Once again, one must note the importance of a meticulous assessment of the entire sympathetic and parasympathetic pathways to search for the cause of this syndrome, particularly in emergencies and when carotid artery dissection is suspected.

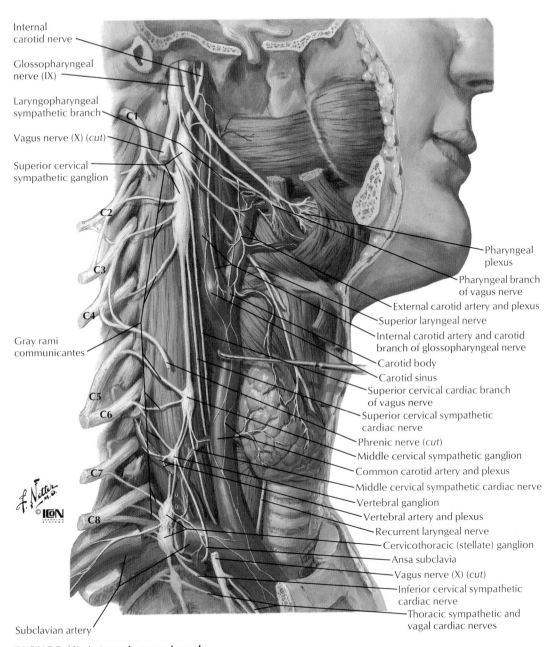

Internal carotid nerve

Glossopharyngeal nerve (IX)

Laryngopharyngeal sympathetic branch

Vagus nerve (X) (*cut*)

Superior cervical sympathetic ganglion

C1

C2

C3

C4

Gray rami communicantes

C5

C6

C7

C8

Subclavian artery

Pharyngeal plexus

Pharyngeal branch of vagus nerve

External carotid artery and plexus

Superior laryngeal nerve

Internal carotid artery and carotid branch of glossopharyngeal nerve

Carotid body

Carotid sinus

Superior cervical cardiac branch of vagus nerve

Superior cervical sympathetic cardiac nerve

Phrenic nerve (*cut*)

Middle cervical sympathetic ganglion

Common carotid artery and plexus

Middle cervical sympathetic cardiac nerve

Vertebral ganglion

Vertebral artery and plexus

Recurrent laryngeal nerve

Cervicothoracic (stellate) ganglion

Ansa subclavia

Vagus nerve (X) (*cut*)

Inferior cervical sympathetic cardiac nerve

Thoracic sympathetic and vagal cardiac nerves

FIGURE IX Autonomic nerves in neck

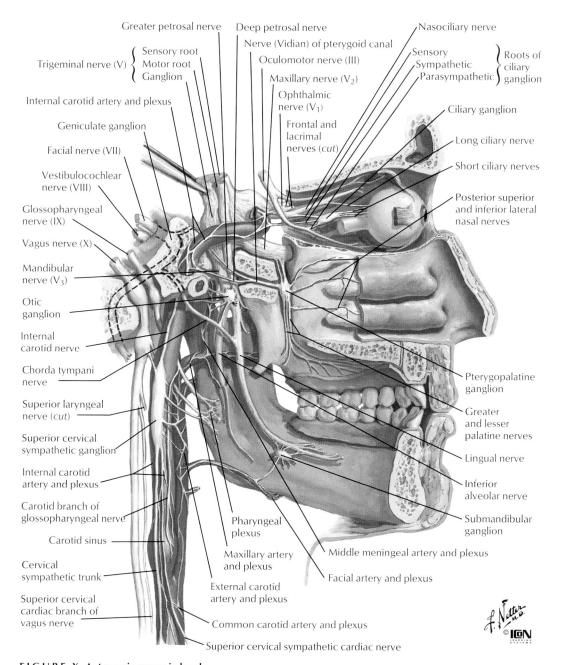

Greater petrosal nerve

Deep petrosal nerve

Nerve (Vidian) of pterygoid canal

Nasociliary nerve

Trigeminal nerve (V) { Sensory root / Motor root / Ganglion

Oculomotor nerve (III)

Maxillary nerve (V₂)

Sensory / Sympathetic / Parasympathetic } Roots of ciliary ganglion

Internal carotid artery and plexus

Ophthalmic nerve (V₁)

Ciliary ganglion

Geniculate ganglion

Frontal and lacrimal nerves (*cut*)

Long ciliary nerve

Facial nerve (VII)

Short ciliary nerves

Vestibulocochlear nerve (VIII)

Posterior superior and inferior lateral nasal nerves

Glossopharyngeal nerve (IX)

Vagus nerve (X)

Mandibular nerve (V₃)

Otic ganglion

Internal carotid nerve

Chorda tympani nerve

Pterygopalatine ganglion

Superior laryngeal nerve (*cut*)

Greater and lesser palatine nerves

Superior cervical sympathetic ganglion

Lingual nerve

Internal carotid artery and plexus

Inferior alveolar nerve

Carotid branch of glossopharyngeal nerve

Submandibular ganglion

Carotid sinus

Pharyngeal plexus

Cervical sympathetic trunk

Maxillary artery and plexus

Middle meningeal artery and plexus

Superior cervical cardiac branch of vagus nerve

External carotid artery and plexus

Facial artery and plexus

Common carotid artery and plexus

Superior cervical sympathetic cardiac nerve

FIGURE X Autonomic nerves in head

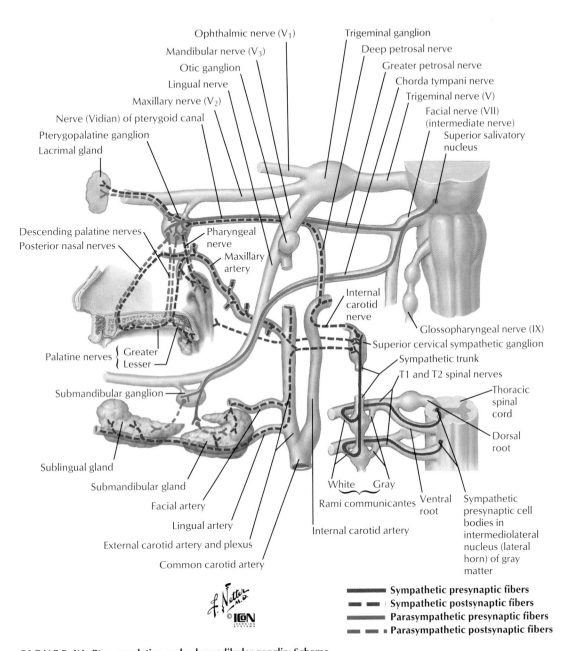

Ophthalmic nerve (V$_1$)
Mandibular nerve (V$_3$)
Otic ganglion
Lingual nerve
Maxillary nerve (V$_2$)
Nerve (Vidian) of pterygoid canal
Pterygopalatine ganglion
Lacrimal gland

Trigeminal ganglion
Deep petrosal nerve
Greater petrosal nerve
Chorda tympani nerve
Trigeminal nerve (V)
Facial nerve (VII)
(intermediate nerve)
Superior salivatory
nucleus

Descending palatine nerves
Posterior nasal nerves
Pharyngeal nerve
Maxillary artery

Internal carotid nerve

Glossopharyngeal nerve (IX)
Superior cervical sympathetic ganglion
Sympathetic trunk
T1 and T2 spinal nerves

Palatine nerves { Greater
Lesser

Submandibular ganglion

Thoracic spinal cord

Dorsal root

Sublingual gland
Submandibular gland
Facial artery
Lingual artery
External carotid artery and plexus
Common carotid artery

White   Gray
Rami communicantes   Ventral root
Internal carotid artery

Sympathetic presynaptic cell bodies in intermediolateral nucleus (lateral horn) of gray matter

▬▬▬▬ Sympathetic presynaptic fibers
▬ ▬ ▬ Sympathetic postsynaptic fibers
▬▬▬▬ Parasympathetic presynaptic fibers
▬ ▬ ▬ Parasympathetic postsynaptic fibers

FIGURE XI Pterygopalatine and submandibular ganglia: Schema

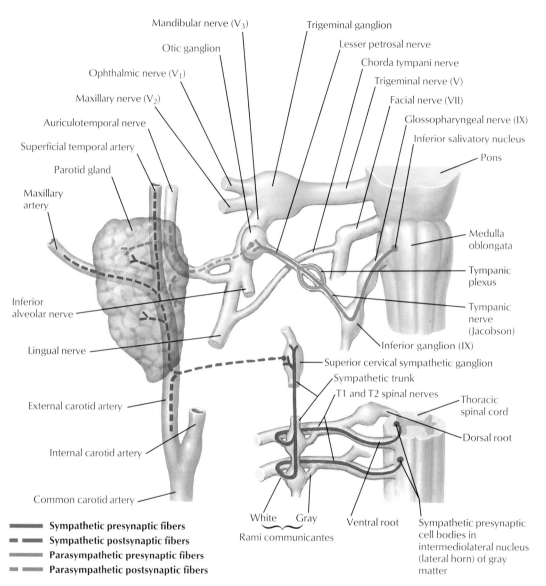

Mandibular nerve (V₃)
Otic ganglion
Ophthalmic nerve (V₁)
Maxillary nerve (V₂)
Auriculotemporal nerve
Superficial temporal artery
Parotid gland
Maxillary artery
Inferior alveolar nerve
Lingual nerve
External carotid artery
Internal carotid artery
Common carotid artery

Trigeminal ganglion
Lesser petrosal nerve
Chorda tympani nerve
Trigeminal nerve (V)
Facial nerve (VII)
Glossopharyngeal nerve (IX)
Inferior salivatory nucleus
Pons
Medulla oblongata
Tympanic plexus
Tympanic nerve (Jacobson)
Inferior ganglion (IX)
Superior cervical sympathetic ganglion
Sympathetic trunk
T1 and T2 spinal nerves
Thoracic spinal cord
Dorsal root

White   Gray
Rami communicantes

Ventral root

Sympathetic presynaptic cell bodies in intermediolateral nucleus (lateral horn) of gray matter

━━━ **Sympathetic presynaptic fibers**
╺ ━ **Sympathetic postsynaptic fibers**
━━━ **Parasympathetic presynaptic fibers**
╺ ━ **Parasympathetic postsynaptic fibers**

FIGURE XII Otis ganglion: Schema

Atlas SW. *Magnetic resonance imaging of the brain and spine.* 2nd ed. Philadelphia: Lippincott-Raven;1996:1675.

Boecher-Schwarz HG, Bruehl K, Kessel G, Guenthner M, Perneczky A, Stoeter P. Sensitivity and specificity or MRI in the diagnosis of neuromuscular compression in patients with trigeminal neuralgia. A correlation of MRI and surgical findings. *Neuroradiologie* 1998;40:88–95.

Bossy J. *Neuroanatomie.* Springer Verlag, 1990, 475 p.

Bourjat P, Speeg-Schatz, Kahn JL. *Imagerie oculo-orbitaire.* Masson; 2000:154.

Bourjat P, Veillon F. *Imagerie radiologique tête et cou.* Vigot; 1995:524.

Brunereau L, Gobin YP, Meder JF, Cognard C, Tubianaa JM, Merland JJ. Intracranial dural arteriovenous fistulas with spinal venous drainage: relation between clinical presentation and angiographic findings. *AJNR Am J Neuroradiol* 1996;17: 1549–1554.

Cabanis EA, Bourgeouis H, IBA-Zizen MT. *L'imagerie en ophtalmologie.* Masson; 1996:761.

Cambier J, Masson M, Dehem R. *Neurologie.* Masson; 1995:599.

Casselman JW, Kuhweide R, Ampe W, Meeus L, Steyaert L. Pathology of the membranous labyrinth: Comparison of T1, T2, and Gd-enhanced T1 weighted spin echo imaging and 3 DFT-CISS imaging. *AJNR Am J Neuroradiol* 1993;14:47–57.

Casselman JW, Officier FE, et al. Aplasia and hypoplasia of the vestibulocochlear nerve: Diagnostic with MR imaging. *Radiology* 1997;202: 773–781.

Cognard C, Gobin YP, Pierot L, et al. Cerebral dural arteriovenous fistulas: Clinical and angiographic correlation with a revised classification of venous drainage. *Radiology* 1995;194:671–680.

Davis SB, Mathews VP, Williams DW. Masticator muscle enhancement in subacute denervation atrophy. *AJNR Am J Neuroradiol* 1995;16:1290–1294.

Feneis H. *Répertoire illustré d'anatomie humaine.* Prodim medsi; 1986:485.

Ginsburg LE, Pruett SK, Chen MY, et al. Skull base foramina of the middle cranial fossa reasseament of normal variation with hight resolution CT. *AJNR Am J Neuroradiol* 1994;15:283–291.

Harnsberger HR. *Handbook of Head and Neck Imaging.* 2nd ed. St Louis: Mosby;1995:556.

Harrison TR. *Principes de medicine interne.* 12th ed. Flammarion; 1992:1173.

Kamina P. *Dictionnaire atlas d'anatomie.* Maloine; 1983:1843.

Lang J. *Clinical anatomy of the nose, nasal cavity and para nasal sinuses.* Theime; 1989:144.

Lapresle J, Fernandez-Manchola I, Lasjaunias P. L'atteinte trigeminale sensitive au cours de la paralysie faciale peripherique essentielle. Nouv Presse Med; 1980;9:291–293.

Lapresle J, Lasjaunias P. Cranial nerve ischemic arterial syndromes. *Brain* 1986;109:207–215.

Lasjaunias P, Doyon D, Edouard A. Les paralysies faciales périphériques post-embolisation : Rapport sur un cas, discussion, prévention. *Ann oto-laryng* 1978;95:595–602.

Lasjaunias P, Berenstein A, Ter Brugge LKG. *Surgical neuro-angiography.* 2nd ed. Springer; 2001.

Leblanc A. *Les nerfs crâniens.* 2nd ed. Springer; 1995:300.

Leblanc A. *Système nerveux encéphalo-périphérique vascularisation, anatomie, imagerie.* Springer; 2001:438.

Levy C, Laissy JP, Raveau V, Amarenco P, Servois V, Bousser MG, Tubiana JM. Carotid and vertebral artery dissections: Three dimension time-of-flight MR angiography and MR imaging versus conventional angiography. *Radiology* 1994;190:97–103.

Libersa C. *Etude de la vascularisation artérielle des nerfs crâniens et du paquet acoustico-facial.* Sautai et Fils Lille; 1951.

Magnan J, Chays A, Girard N. Syndrome de compression des nerfs crâniens. In Pathologie vasculaire en ORL, rapport de la Société française d'ORL et de chirurgie de la face et du cou, Romanet Ph, Paris; Septembre 2000.

Magnan J, Chays A, Caces F, Locatelli P. Hemifacial spasm: Endoscopic vascular decompression. Acoustic neuroma and skull base surgery. 1995;557–564.

Magnan J, Chays A, Broder L, Brusso M, El Garem H, Girard N, RAYBAUD C. Le traitement des conflits artère-nerfs dans l'angle ponto-cérébelleux. *Radiologie J CEPUR* 1999;19(2):63–72.

Majoie CBL, Verberrten B, Dol JA, Peeters FL. Trigeminal neuropathy: Evaluation with MR imaging. *Radiographics* 1995;15:795–811.

Majoie CBL, Hulsmans FJH, Verbeeten B Jr, Castelijns JA, van Beek EJR, Valk J, Bosch AD. Trigeminal neuralgia: Comparison of two MR imaging techniques in the demonstration of neuromuscular contact. *Radiology* 1997;204:455–460.

Marsot-Dupuch K. Imagerie de l'oreille interne: Aspect normal et pathologique. *EMC Otorhino-laryngologie* 20-047-A-10, 1999:16.

Marsot-Dupuch K. Pulsatile and non-pulsatile tinnitus: A systemic approach. *Semin Ultrasound CT MRI* 2001;22(3):250–270.

Marsot-Dupuch K. Imagerie des nerfs crâniens. 60e Journées du CER Saint-Antoine.

Netter FH. *Cranial nerves in the Ciba Collection.* Vol. 21, Part 1. 1991:92–109.

Raybaud CH, Girard N, Poncet M, Chays A, Caces F, Magnan J. L'imagerie actuelle des conflits vasculo-nerveux de l'angle ponto-cérébelleux. *Rev Laryngol Otol Rhinol* 1995;116(2):99–103.

Russo C, Smoker WRT, Weissman JL. MR appearance of trigeminal and hypoglosseal motor denervation. *AJNR Am J Neuroradiol* 1997;18:1375–1383.

Samii M, Inaetta PJ. *The Cranial Nerves.* Springer; 1981.

Sismanis A. Pulsatile tinnitus. A 15 year experience. *Am J Otol* 1998;19:472–477.

Sismanis A, Hughes GB, Abedi E, et al. Otologic symptoms and findings of the pseudotumor cerebri syndrome: A preliminary report. *Otolaryngol Head Neck Surg* 1985;93:398–402.

Sismanis A, Smoker WRK. Pulsatile tinnitus: Recent advances in diagnosis. *Laryngoscope* 1994;104:681–688.

Tien RD, Wilkins RH. MRI delineation of the vertebral-basilar system in patients with hemifacial spasm and trigeminal neuralgia. *AJNR Am J Neuroradiol* 1993;14:34–36.

van der Knaap MS, Valk J. *Magnetic resonance of myeline, myelination and myelin disorders.* Springer; 1995.

Williams LS, Schmalfussim, Sistrom CL, Inoue T, Tanaka R, Seoane ER, Mancuso AA. MR imaging of the trigeminal ganglion, nerve and the perineural vascular plexus: Normal appearance and variants with correlation to cadaver specimens. *AJNR Am J Neuroradiol* 2003;24:1317–1323.

Note: Page numbers followed by *f* and *t* indicate figures and tables, respectively.